Teaching Made Easy

Teaching Made Easy

A MANUAL FOR HEALTH PROFESSIONALS

Third Edition

KAY MOHANNA
ELIZABETH COTTRELL
DAVID WALL

and

RUTH CHAMBERS

Radcliffe Publishing
Oxford • New York

Radcliffe Publishing Ltd
18 Marcham Road
Abingdon
Oxon OX14 1AA
United Kingdom

www.radcliffepublishing.com

Electronic catalogue and worldwide online ordering facility.

The paper used for the text pages of this book is FSC certified. FSC (The Forest Stewardship Council) is an international network to promote responsible management of the world's forests.

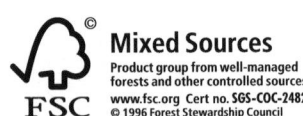

Mixed Sources
Product group from well-managed forests and other controlled sources
www.fsc.org Cert no. SGS-COC-2482
© 1996 Forest Stewardship Council

Typeset by Pindar NZ, Auckland, New Zealand
Printed and bound by TJI Digital, Padstow, Cornwall, UK

Contents

Preface

This is the third edition of *Teaching Made Easy*. Substantial changes have been made based on feedback obtained from both experienced and student teachers.

Teaching Made Easy is for those who are learning to become healthcare teachers and those who are new to teaching roles. However, it will provide structure, support and guidance on maintaining standards for novice and experienced teachers. Furthermore, the latest edition of this book will help you to improve the effectiveness of your teaching, through improving the delivery and organisation of education events, and to demonstrate this effectiveness. The tips that are provided about the management of difficult situations encourage sensitive and constructive guidance of learners.

Teaching Made Easy now places less emphasis on the UK healthcare system alone. The book is widely read and respected worldwide, so this current edition has been developed for use by international readers. The content is also more relevant to and inclusive of all healthcare disciplines.

The content of previous editions has been reorganised to ensure more intuitive placement of information. Key points are now highlighted by the inclusion of *Tips from experienced teachers* in each chapter.

To address changing times, new chapters reflect contemporary concepts and key approaches. The new chapters are 'Starting out and developing as a teacher' (Chapter 1), 'Developing your teaching style and techniques' (Chapter 6), 'Curriculum: constructing a programme for learning' (Chapter 7), 'E-learning and virtual learning environments' (Chapter 9), 'Teaching in ambulatory care settings' (Chapter 10), 'Writing educational materials' (Chapter 12) and 'Leadership training' (Chapter 19).

We are proud of this latest edition, and feel that it builds upon an already well received and useful resource for both new and experienced healthcare teachers.

Kay Mohanna
Elizabeth Cottrell
David Wall
Ruth Chambers
November 2010

About the authors

Kay Mohanna (UK) is a senior lecturer at Keele University Medical School, where she is Director of Postgraduate Medicine and is responsible for the Masters in Medical Education award. She chairs the Midland Faculty of the Royal College of General Practitioners (RCGP), and sits on the Central RCGP Council and Postgraduate School of General Practice at the West Midlands Strategic Health Authority. Until recently she was Associate Dean for the introduction of the new Member of the RCGP (MRCGP) assessment process and educational supervision training in the West Midlands.

Her research interests have included risk communication and informed consent, particularly with regard to research in pregnant women, teaching styles assessment and study skills support. She is author or co-author of 13 books, including the official RCGP resource for specialist training in general practice.

Elizabeth Cottrell (UK) is an Academic Clinical Fellow in General Practice Specialty Training at the University Hospital of North Staffordshire NHS Trust and Keele University. Although her academic work at present is research based, she has pursued her interest in medical education by undertaking a *Teaching the Teachers* course, and through her involvement in organising and providing career support for medical students at Keele University following the writing of *The Medical Student Career Handbook*, which is now in its second edition.

David Wall (UK) is Deputy Regional Postgraduate Dean in the West Midlands Deanery and Honorary Professor of medical education at Staffordshire University. He has been a general practitioner in Four Oaks, Sutton Coldfield for 30 years, having started there in 1974. He obtained a Diploma in Medical Education from the University of Dundee in 1996, and a Masters degree in 1998. He was awarded a PhD in Education from the University of Birmingham in 2007. His main work in the Deanery is with doctors and dentists in difficulty, educational research (including educational climate, selection of trainees, and education being fit for purpose) and faculty development.

Ruth Chambers (UK) has been a family doctor for 30 years and is Honorary Professor of primary care at Staffordshire University. She has undertaken a diverse range of teaching roles in the course of her career, including plenary presentations to thousands of people, regular lectures, small group work and interactive workshops, one-to-one tutorials and ad-hoc teaching opportunities. Her previous research interests have focused on self-care, effective ways of working, stress in healthcare professionals, and many other health-related themes in various healthcare settings.

Ruth often works with the Royal College of General Practitioners, the Department of Health and other healthcare organisations on various projects. Most of her teaching and quality initiatives have related to improving performance and effective ways of working in the health service. She has written around 70 books, mainly for healthcare professionals, but two of her most recently published titles are for the general public, on heart disease and back pain.

Helen Batty (Canada) is a Full Professor in the Department of Family and Community Medicine at the University of Toronto. She is the Founding Director of the Academic Fellowship and the Graduate Studies programmes for the Department, including the Clinical Teacher Certificate, the INTAPT (Interprofessional Teaching and Learning) Programme, the Enhanced Clinical Fellowship and the new Master of Science in Community Health (MScCH) Health Professions Teacher Education degree programme. In 2005 she won the National Award for Outstanding Contribution to Faculty Development from the Association of Faculties of Medicine of Canada (AFMC). In 2008 she won the University of Toronto's President's Teaching Award, the highest teaching honour in the institution recognising sustained excellence in teaching, research in teaching, and the integration of teaching and research. She practises at Women's College Hospital. Since her faculty appointment in 1975, she has taught undergraduate, postgraduate and graduate learners, community clinicians and faculty in multiple healthcare professions. Helen has recently been awarded the 2010 CAME-Ian Hart Award, a national Canadian award for distinguished contribution to medical education.

Stephen Bostock (UK) is Head of the Learning Development Unit at Keele University, and coordinates the enhancement of learning and teaching institutionally, including all staff development for teaching, strategic management of the e-learning environment, innovation awards and teaching excellence awards. He is course director of the postgraduate Certificate in Teaching and Learning with Technology programme and of the MA in Learning and Teaching in Higher Education. In 2004 he won a university Award for Learning and Teaching Excellence, and in 2009 he won a National Teaching Fellowship. A Fellow of the Staff and Educational Development Association, he is Chair of its Professional Development Framework Committee, and accredits programmes at institutions internationally.

Mike Deighan (UK) is a GP in Worcester and Head of the Postgraduate School of General Practice in the West Midlands Deanery. He was one of the authors of the RCGP Curriculum for GP Specialty Training. As well as being an enthusiastic GP trainer, he teaches postgraduate students at the University of Birmingham and the University of Keele. In addition to teaching, learning and curriculum, he has a keen academic interest in assessment. He is an assessor for the MRCGP clinical skills assessment and is an external examiner for MRCGP International.

Acknowledgements

This third edition of *Teaching Made Easy* has been informed by feedback that we have gratefully received from colleagues working as teachers in the healthcare professions and student-teacher users of the book – in particular, dozens of students of medical education who sent us their observations, and Dr Sally Chambers, Keele University Teaching Fellow, and Specialist Registrar in Geriatric Medicine, who provided multiple suggestions for changes to the book. The experiences of international healthcare students have provided invaluable insights into desirable and undesirable qualities of teachers (*see* Chapter 1), and we thank Kinjal Banerjee, Rob Chambers, Emma Stephens and Akshay Sharma for their time and thoughts.

We are especially grateful for the hard work and time given to this third edition by three additional authors, namely Helen Batty (Chapter 10 and the *Teaching practical skills* section of Chapter 8), Stephen Bostock (Chapter 9) and Mike Deighan (Chapter 7). The specific and extensive experience of these authors has significantly increased the quality of the information that we present to you.

Professor Gerald Grow has generously given permission for his *stages of self-direction model* to be reproduced together with his own illustrations in Chapter 5. We would urge you to visit his website (www.longleaf.net/ggrow) for further insights.

As the behaviourist BF Skinner said, 'Education is what remains when what was taught has been forgotten.' Many of the insights that we have used in this book came from our own teachers in our study of education. They are things that have worked for us. It would be impossible to name all of the influences, even if we could tease out who had taught us what. If you recognise your words in our work, you were a good teacher.

Thank you.

Glossary of terms

Clinical governance: a system being implemented throughout the NHS which will assure the public of minimum standards, and encourage good practice and the delivery of cost-effective care by the NHS workforce as a whole.

Coaching: the process of motivating, encouraging and helping an individual to improve his or her skills, knowledge and attitudes in a framework of goal setting and achievement.

Continuing medical education: the learning of core knowledge and skills in a specialty area; this can be synonymous with *continuing professional development* in some countries.

Continuing professional development: 'a process of lifelong learning for all individuals and teams which enables professionals to expand and fulfil their potential and which also meets the needs of patients and delivers the health and healthcare priorities of the NHS.'[1]

Mentor: an experienced, highly regarded, empathetic person who guides another individual in the development of his or her reflection, learning, and personal, professional and career development.

Mentoring: 'an ancient process of learning facilitation by mutual professional support, traditionally given by a senior to a junior colleague.'[1]

Peer appraisal: the process by which colleagues identify and constructively discuss each other's strengths, weaknesses and learning needs within a supportive environment.

Personal development plan: a document describing an individual's learning objectives, the processes by which these objectives are defined and expected to be achieved, and how the achievement of these objectives will be evaluated.

Portfolio: a collection of evidence demonstrating how personal learning has been fulfilled.

Reflection: the process whereby people actively deliberate on their performance or the care that they deliver, and identify their strengths and weaknesses (either as individuals or in groups).

Revalidation: a compulsory episodic affirmation that a doctor continues to be fit to practise.

Training: a process which is planned to facilitate learning so that people can become effective in carrying out aspects of their work.

REFERENCE

1   Chief Medical Officer. *A Review of Continuing Professional Development in General Practice.* London: Department of Health; 1998.

List of abbreviations

AAMC	Association of American Medical Colleges
AoME	Academy of Medical Educators
CHD	coronary heart disease
CME	continuing medical education
CoPMeD	Conference of Postgraduate Medical Deans
CPD	continuing professional development
DOPS	direct observation of procedural skills
ENB	English National Board
EWTD	European Working Time Directive
FMRAC	Federation of Medical Regulatory Authorities of Canada
GMC	General Medical Council
MCQ	multiple choice question
MSF	multi-source feedback
NCAS	National Clinical Assessment Service
NHS	National Health Service
NLC	National Leadership Council
NLP	neurolinguistic programming
NMC	Nursing and Midwifery Council
OSCE	objective structured clinical examination
PAL	peer-assisted learning
PBA	procedure-based assessment
PBL	problem-based learning
PDP	personal development plan
PREP	post-registration education and practice
RCGP	Royal College of General Practitioners
RCN	Royal College of Nursing
RCT	randomised controlled trials
SCOPME	Standing Committee on Postgraduate Medical and Dental Education
SSDL	stages of self-directed learning

TERMINOLOGY

Unless otherwise specified, the term 'learner' refers to any of the following: learner, student, trainee, tutee or participant who takes part in a learning programme in order to learn. The term 'teacher' refers to a teacher, trainer, supervisor, educator or tutor who takes part in teaching and facilitating learning.

CHAPTER 1

Starting out and developing as a teacher

Teaching, much like clinical work, requires the appropriate knowledge, skills and attitudes. How you teach is influenced by your innate style, the subject matter and learner group. Some elements of a 'good' teacher may evolve naturally. However, there will always be challenges and room for review, reflection and refinement of your performance.

How do you plan to pursue your interest in teaching healthcare professionals? Opportunities and career choices are not always highly visible. You may not always find someone to provide the advice you need. This chapter guides you to find out more about teaching healthcare professionals and ways in which you can formalise this.

Grasping the appropriate knowledge, skills and attitudes is not enough. You must continually strive to improve these qualities, and must formally demonstrate such improvement. The latter part of this chapter will assist you with doing this.

GAINING EXPERIENCE

Find out more

The first step in embarking on a teaching career is to try it out. The availability of opportunities for gaining additional experience will depend on your current circumstances. However, everyone can reflect on previous teaching experiences. Think about different teaching scenarios – for example, communication skills training, small group work or problem-based learning (PBL). Which teachers did you feel were effective, inspirational or 'good'? Think about previous poor or frustrating teaching experiences. Why do you think this was the case? What could have been done to change this? After reading this book, you may be able to better identify reasons for effective or poor teaching. Box 1.1 lists examples of such reflections from international healthcare students.

BOX 1.1 Students' perspectives on qualities of 'good' and 'poor' teachers

Based on past experiences, learners were asked what elements resulted in a good teaching experience and/or a good teacher. They suggested the following:

- Enthusiasm, a love for the subject.
- A questioning, challenging, patient approach – ensured depth of knowledge rather than mere rote learning.
- Focused, clear aims (outlined at the beginning of the teaching session), concentrating on the main points.
- Good knowledge of and interest in the subject, knowing what the learner needs to know, intelligent, willing to answer questions, experienced.
- Good relationship with learners, approachable, listening, interacting with learners at their level, mutual respect between teacher and learner, showing empathy, understanding and consideration in relation to learners, taking an interest in the learners and their experiences, 'understanding our feelings', being keen to learn from learners.
- Being supportive (e.g. to those who struggle by arranging an extra tutorial, giving additional feedback on submitted work, etc.).
- High level of class participation, trying to make classes interesting, liberal use of teaching aids.
- Going back to basics – 'the teacher made us think the clinical problems through in a logical way, which made us realise that we could work answers out if we followed a logical pattern.'
- Relating the subject back to real life and/or clinical scenarios – 'we could see why each piece of information was important and where it fitted in.'
- A dynamic and adaptable style of teaching, using pictures, PowerPoint, etc. as necessary and appropriate.
- Ability to project voice across a room so that everyone can clearly hear what they are saying.
- Understanding that learners have different knowledge levels, not reacting negatively if learners do not know something, and making sure that learners have learned what they were supposed to learn.

Students' thoughts on what made teaching experiences negative:
- Boring, lack of involvement of learners and/or the teacher talking all the time.
- Uncertain session objectives.
- Running out of time, poor organisation, the teacher being late for the session, the session being held at a bad time of the day, the teaching session being too long and/ or without a break.
- Teaching 'bookish knowledge', repeating exactly what was in books.
- Lack of interest in subject and/or teaching.
- Lack of guidance with assignments.
- 'Us and them' boundaries put in place between tutors and students.
- Poor communication – mumbling when addressing the class, no eye contact, reading off PowerPoint slides.
- Teaching by humiliation – 'making me feel stupid in front of my peers when I couldn't think of an answer.'

- Unnecessary emphasis on minutiae.

Effects of negative teaching experiences on the learner:
- Unable to test understanding or experience learners' opinions, arguments or approaches.
- Frustration.
- Feeling as if time is being wasted and/or there is not much to gain from the teacher. This may lead to the learner not looking forward to, or even not going back to, another teaching session given by the same person.
- Loss of interest, poor attention, clock watching, talking to other learners.
- Lack of respect for the teacher.
- Feeling stupid, losing confidence, and being scared of being wrong in the future.
- Missing out on the subject matter because the learner 'switched off', no or limited learning.
- Being 'put off' the subject.

How learners feel teaching experiences may be improved:
- Teacher interacts with students – for example, by using prompts to open discussion.
- Encouraging learners to participate verbally or with hands-on exercises.
- Changing the way they teach to make it more content relevant and interesting, rather than just 'bookish knowledge'.
- Using a mix of teaching styles – didactic learning, group work, class participation, discussing theory.
- Having a clear structure, being organised, clarifying what the aims and objectives of the session and/or programme are. Sometimes asking learners what their expectations of the session are causes those who are not clear to understand, and enables the teacher to direct the learners to the actual point of the session if they have got this wrong.
- Relating the teaching to clinical scenarios, telling the learners what they need to know both for exams and for clinical practice.
- Ensure that there is enough time for the planned content of the teaching session to be delivered.

Talk with local educationalists about careers options. Either approach current or previous tutors or seek out relevant people from staff lists on university websites to obtain discipline-specific information. General information is available from educational associations and organisations (*see* Box 1.2).

BOX 1.2 Examples of educational associations and organisations

Organisations for healthcare professionals and/or students in general: Association for Health Professional Education (ANZAME, www.anzame.unsw.edu.au), Education Scholar (www.educationscholar.org/index.htm), Health Care Education Association (HCEA, www.hcea-info.org), MedEdCentral (www.mededcentral.org/index.aspx), MedEdWorld (www.mededworld.org), Medical Education Online (MEO, http://med-ed-online.net)

Dentists and/or dental students: American Dental Education Association (ADEA, www.adea.org), Association for Dental Education in Europe (ADEE, www.adee.org), International Federation of Dental Educators and Associations (IFDEA, www.ifdea.org)

Doctors and/or medical students: Academy of Medical Educators (www.medicaleducators.org), Association for the Study of Medical Education (ASME, www.asme.org.uk), International Association for Medical Education in Europe (AMEE, www.amee.org), Society of Teachers of Family Medicine (STFM, www.stfm.org)

Physiotherapists and/or physiotherapy students: International Society of Educators in Physiotherapy (ISEP, www.isep.org.au)

Nurses and/or student nurses: Association of District Nurse Educators (ADNE, www.adne.co.uk), National League for Nursing (NLN, www.nln.org), Professional Nurse Educators Group (PNEG, www.pneg.org)

Midwives: Association for Midwifery Educators (www.associationofmidwiferyeducators.org)

Many healthcare courses now include peer-assisted learning (PAL) initiatives that provide those involved with experience of teaching, experience of being role models for juniors[1] and improved success in studies and exams.[2] PAL initiatives may exist within your university/college, so find out from your tutors. If such initiatives do not exist, consider starting one, as medical students in Sheffield, UK, did when they founded a 'Peer Teaching Society' to facilitate those with an interest in education to develop their skills.[2] National PAL initiatives also exist. For example, Sexpression:UK (www.sexpression.org.uk) involves UK medical students teaching sex education to local secondary school children.

Seek opportunities to understand assessments 'from the other side' by assisting with a station in a practical clinical exam. You will see how learners are marked and the limitations of such examination methods.

Speak with senior faculty staff, express your interest in teaching, and they may direct you to, or create, opportunities to become involved in undergraduate course development, management or delivery. Certain opportunities may only be available to postgraduates, but expressing your interest early on may invite opportunities (e.g. facilitating PBL groups, teaching anatomy, running special interest groups or committees or journal clubs).

Undertake formal training

If you are serious about teaching and would like to formalise this, you should gain a theoretical background and undertake a course or recognised educational qualification in the subject. This will enable you to improve your skills, and will provide good evidence of your commitment and level of attainment when applying for future educational posts. Multiple accredited qualifications exist (*see* Box 1.3). The right one for you will depend upon your discipline/specialty, where you live and/or work and your current level of training. Specific information can be found on the relevant awarding institution's website.

BOX 1.3 Educational qualifications

Healthcare professionals/students in general
- Introductory courses: Teaching the Teachers (individual institutions run these courses differently, so consult local information) and the Dundee *Discovery Courses* (www.dundee.ac.uk/meded/frames/courses/Discovery.html)
- Higher degrees (Certificate/Diploma/Masters/PhD):
  - *Medical education*: the Foundation for Advancement of International Medical Education and Research (FAIMER) has collated details of institutions that host Masters programmes in medical education (www.faimer.org/resources/mastersmeded.html)
  - Adult education or learning and teaching or education: not specific for educating healthcare professionals, and often undertaken by non-medical educators as the availability of profession-specific educational higher degrees is limited
- Other: *Education Scholar* (www.educationscholar.org/index.htm)

Doctors/medical students
- *Scaling the Heights* (www.scalingtheheights.co.uk), *Essential Skills in Medical Education* (http://esmeprogramme.org) accredited by AMEE

Physiotherapists/physiotherapy students
- *Clinical Educators* courses: see the UK Chartered Society of Physiotherapy website (search for accreditation of clinical educators on www.csp.org.uk)

Midwives/midwifery students
- *Programmes of Preparation for Supervisors of Midwives* (UK) (www.nmc-uk.org) *Preceptorship courses* (Canada, New Zealand) (www.midwiferyjunction.co.nz/midwives/become-preceptor-midwife)

Nurses/student nurses
- *Master of Science in Nursing Education* (USA): see *Certification for Nurse Educators* (USA) (www.nln.org/facultycertification/index.htm)

Radiographers/radiography students
- *Practice Educator Accreditation Scheme* (www.sor.org/public/practice-educator/index.htm)

Occupational therapists/occupational therapy students
- Accreditation of Practice Placement Educators (APPLE) (www.cot.co.uk/MainWebSite/C0a8e98af2.aspx?Map=7D4DDEA421683295918B276E284FF2E6)

Look for formal roles

Depending upon your discipline, the country in which you work and your level of experience and qualifications, a large range of formal educational posts are available (*see* Box 1.4). Further details can be found in the resources listed in *Further Reading*, or from the appropriate professional organisation websites.

BOX 1.4 Formal educational posts

Integrated academic and clinical training schemes: when the importance of streamlining academic and clinical training was recognised, integrated training schemes were developed. For example, the UK National Institute for Health Research (NIHR) Integrated Academic Training scheme funds posts for trainee doctors that enable them to continue training in their chosen specialty while undertaking basic training in the academic field. A few of these schemes are education (rather than research) based (see www.nihrtcc.nhs.uk/intetacatrain).

Mentor, careers counsellor or coach: *see* Chapter 18.

Clinical and/or educational supervisory roles:
- Doctors – educational/clinical supervisors, trainers or faculty for junior doctors.
- Physiotherapists – clinical educators.
- Nurses – practice educators, preceptors, clinical supervisor.
- Midwives – supervisor of midwives (UK), midwife preceptor (Canada, USA, New Zealand).

Within training and/or postgraduate continuing professional development organisations, deaneries and/or universities: examples of teaching posts are Teaching Fellow, Lecturer, Lecturer Practitioner, Lead Midwife for Education, Clinical Nurse Educator, Professor, Dean and Programme Director. Such roles may involve the following responsibilities to varying extents: developing courses and curricula, teaching students/ postgraduate trainees/fully qualified professionals, evaluating teaching and learning and devising assessments. Some posts may also require you to undertake formal research, including writing grant proposals.

Within professional organisations: specialty-specific professional bodies and/or educational organisations offer formal posts that enable you to develop your field of education using a top-down approach (e.g. committee positions, being an appraiser or quality assessor).

REVIEWING PERFORMANCE

In order to achieve and maintain good teaching practice, you must review your performance.

> Good quality preparation of supervisors and ongoing assessment of their performance is essential to effective supervision.[3]

So how do you do this? Your performance can be reviewed through:
➤ self-evaluation
➤ peer- or teaching evaluation (*see* Chapter 16)
➤ learner evaluation (*see* Chapter 16)
➤ multi-source feedback (*see* Chapter 13).

Certain evaluations in some posts are compulsory. However, if they are not, you should still seek feedback to facilitate your development. Review of your performance will highlight areas that are in need of improvement and those in which you excel. This knowledge can be developed into a personal development plan (PDP) (see below).

Self-rate your teaching competences

Reflecting on your skills and progress and undertaking a realistic assessment of your teaching are crucial for ongoing development. By gathering evidence and reflecting on why your teaching sessions have gone exceptionally well (or were a disaster) you can use this information, along with the advice in the rest of this book, to address your personal development areas and to refine your teaching techniques and styles.

Creating a personal development plan (PDP)

Once you are armed with your strengths, weaknesses and areas for further development, you can plan how you will address these. PDPs allow for variations in learning style, personality, experience, interests and job requirements. An effective PDP consists of:

➤ identification of your weaknesses in knowledge, skills or attitudes
➤ specification of topics for learning as a result of changes in your role, your responsibilities, and the organisation
➤ a description of how you identified your learning needs
➤ prioritisation and setting of your learning needs and associated goals
➤ justification of your selection of learning goals
➤ a description of how you will achieve your goals and over what time period
➤ a description of how you will evaluate learning outcomes.

Many healthcare professionals are required to maintain PDPs for managing their personal learning. However, these should not be completed in isolation. Teachers should guide learners through educational conversation, or formative appraisal, to ensure careful and accurate review and well-defined, realistic, achievable and necessary goals.

To assist in the development of a clinical and/or educational PDP, learning objectives must be appropriate and the plan must be clear (*see* Boxes 1.5 and 1.6).[4]

BOX 1.5 How to ensure that PDP learning objectives are appropriate: be SMART[4]

Learning objectives should be:
• Specific
• Measurable
• Achievable
• Relevant
• Time-bounded.

BOX 1.6 The four key elements of a clear plan for learning objectives[4]

1 Statement of the development need.
2 Explanation of how the development need will be addressed (the action to be taken and the resources required).
3 Date by which the goal will be achieved.
4 The intended outcome of the goal.

TABLE 1.1 Framework of an educational needs analysis that is relevant to your current service post

Stage 1: Where are you now? What are your roles and responsibilities? What do you need to know? What skills do you need?

Examples of components and topics that might be relevant for a healthcare professional in a particular post assessing their education needs with respect to their service commitments:

Knowledge	Political awareness	Attitudes	Skills	Aspirations	Context	Legal requirements
Clinical	Policy	To other disciplines	Teamworking	Career	Settings	Health and safety
Information	Priorities	To patients	Communication	Transferable skills	Population	Employment
Resources	Fashions	To lifelong learning	IT capability	Teacher	Networks	Revalidation
Experts	Change	Cultural	Organisational development	Promotion	Organisation's priorities	Safe practice
Best practice			Specialisms	Organisation's mission/vision	Team relationships	
			Competent practitioner		Historical service patterns	

Stage 2: Where do you want to be?

Stage 3: What are your learning needs?

Stage 4: Prioritise your learning needs.

Stage 5: What essential and desirable objectives will you focus on?

Stage 6: What 'tools' (e.g. skills, resources, qualifications, opportunities) do you have?

Stage 7: What 'tools' do you need?

Stage 8: How and when are you going to fulfil your learning objectives?

Stage 9: How will you know when you have achieved your objectives?

Once you have decided your learning goals and priorities, you could check out whether they are appropriate by completing an education, training and development pro forma as in the example in Box 1.7.

Table 1.1 shows a model that can be used to assess educational needs with regard to service needs. Educational needs encompass the context and culture and the knowledge and skills relating to any particular role or responsibility. Add subheadings for categories of knowledge, skill or competence needs that apply to the post in question. Published checklist tools can be used as prompts to inform your lists of topics.[5,6]

Once you have a PDP, you must achieve the specified objectives. A PDP is a dynamic document, and it requires regular review and updating, at least annually, as you achieve the agreed objectives and identify new learning needs. Early in your clinical and educational career you should review your PDP more than once a year, as your needs change rapidly. While undertaking your PDP objectives, gather evidence that each of the objectives has been met, reflect on how you have achieved them, and make a note of further learning objectives that have arisen and how each has changed your practice.

BOX 1.7 Example of an education, training or development activity pro forma

1   How have you identified your learning need(s)?

    a Healthcare system requirement ☐   f New to post ☐

    b Local business plan ☐   g Individual decision ☐

    c Legal mandatory requirement ☐   h Patient feedback ☐

    d Job requirement ☐   i Other ☐

    e Appraisal need ☐

    ....

2   Have you discussed or planned your learning needs with anyone else?

    Yes ☐   No ☐   If so, who?   ....

3   What are the learning need(s) and/or objective(s) in terms of:

    Knowledge: What new information do you hope to gain to help you to do this?

    ....

    Skills: What should you be able to do differently as a result of undertaking this development?

    ....

    Behaviour/professional practice: How will this impact on the way you then do things?

    ....

4   Details and date of desired development activity:

    ....

5   Details and dates of any previous training and/or experience you have had in this area:

    ....

6   What is your current performance in this area against the requirements of your job?

    Need significant development in ☐   Need some development in this ☐
    this area   area

    Satisfactory in this area ☐   Do well in this area ☐

7   Level of job relevance that this area has to your role and responsibilities:

Has no relevance to job   ☐   Has some relevance to job   ☐

Relevant to job   ☐   Very relevant to job   ☐

Essential to job   ☐

Describe what aspect of your job, and how the proposed education/training, is relevant:

....

8   Do you require additional support to identify a suitable   Yes ☐   No ☐
    development activity?

What do you need?

9   Describe the differences or improvements for you, your practice and/or healthcare
    organisation as a result of undertaking this activity:

....

10 Determine the priority of your proposed educational/training activity:

Urgent   ☐   High   ☐   Medium   ☐   Low   ☐

11 Describe how the proposed activity will meet your learning needs rather than any other
    type of course or training on the topic:

....

12 If you had a free choice, would you want to learn this? Yes/No

If **not**, why not? (please circle all that apply):

Waste of time

Have already done it

Not relevant to my work or career goals

Other

If **yes**, what reasons are most important to you? (put them in rank order):

Improve my performance

Increase my knowledge

Get promotion

Just interested

Be better than my colleagues

Do a more interesting job

Be more confident

It will help me

Gathering supporting information and demonstrating achievements and competence

How do you provide evidence of your activities, achievements and competences? Development and maintenance of a contemporary and comprehensive portfolio can achieve this, but first we must understand what competence is.

Competence is a person's ability to perform, and their competences are their total capability (what they can do, which is not necessarily what they actually do). An appropriate definition of 'competence' is:

> the state of having the knowledge, judgement, skills, energy, experience and motivation required to respond adequately to the demands of one's professional responsibilities.[7]

The measurement of competence may be based on three levels of expertise:[8]

➤ aware
➤ competent
➤ expert.

Demonstrating competence through a personal portfolio

A portfolio is a compendium of evidence of your learning, practice and maintenance of standards. How you present this evidence depends upon the purpose of your portfolio. All teachers and learners should maintain a portfolio to demonstrate learning that has occurred. Often the PDP is a good starting point for a portfolio, as it highlights the ongoing development of learning objectives and your plans for improvement. A portfolio can be used to obtain credits for prior learning with higher degree courses, or to prove experience and competence in the future. Finally, your portfolio might form the basis of professional revalidation (see below).

Portfolio-based learning involves the following steps:[9]

➤ identifying significant experiences to serve as important sources of learning
➤ reflecting on the learning that arose from those experiences
➤ demonstrating that learning has been put into practice
➤ analysing the portfolio and identifying further learning needs and ways in which these needs can be met.

As a personal document, a portfolio will have a varied content, which may include some or all of the following:[10-12]

➤ an outline of your current post, responsibilities, aspirations and intermediate to long-term goals
➤ workload logs
➤ case descriptions
➤ evidence of continuing professional development (*see* Chapter 3) (e.g. certificates of attendance, reflection on what has been learned and how your practice will change as a result)
➤ audiovisual examples of your practice (e.g. teaching/presentations given)
➤ patient and/or learner satisfaction surveys
➤ research surveys
➤ audit projects

➤ publications
➤ report of a change or innovation (e.g. in curricula/course design, assessment)
➤ commentaries on published literature or books
➤ records of critical incidents, complaints and learning points (*see* Chapter 5)
➤ an outline of formal teaching sessions with reference to clinical work or other supporting information (e.g. self-, peer and/or learner evaluations, reflections on teaching experiences, whether the style/methods were appropriate for the learners/content/situation)
➤ a summary of your learners' outcomes compared with those of others.

Analysis of experiences and learning opportunities should show demonstrable learning outcomes and resulting educational or developmental needs. Learners may be guided by a mentor as they compile and analyse the material in their portfolio to obtain another perspective that challenges them to think more deeply about their own attitudes, knowledge or beliefs. Much of the learning emanating from a portfolio comes from individual reflection and self-critique.

To ensure that your portfolio demonstrates the standards to which you must work, you must explicitly link the expected standards and your achievement of, or work towards, those standards. Professional educational bodies have published such standards. For example, the Academy of Medical Educators (AoME; www.medicaleducators. org) has produced a framework for those teaching UK medical students and doctors to assist with the demonstration of expertise and achievements in medical education. These standards are subdivided into six themes:[13]

1 values of medical educators
2 educational scholarship (*see* Box 1.8)
3 teaching and supporting learners
4 assessment of and feedback to learners
5 design and planning of learning activities
6 educational management and leadership.

BOX 1.8 Elements of educational scholarship as defined by AoME[13]

- Theoretical base of medical education
- Evidence base of medical education
- Contribution to educational literature
- Critical analysis and evaluation of the evidence base
- Educational research methods
- Educational and information technologies

All of the themes are relevant to your professional development. Graded levels of achievement assist teachers to improve their practice and standards in a stepwise progression. These standards can be generalised and are useful for healthcare teachers worldwide.

Expectations of teachers across different healthcare disciplines are similar (*see* Box 1.9). Table 1.2 shows a simplified version of how expected standards can be mapped to evidence, and this can be generalised across specialties and educational posts.

BOX 1.9 The Chartered Society of Physiotherapy's expectations of physiotherapy clinical educators[14]

The clinical educator should provide evidence that they are able to:
- describe the role and identify the attributes of the effective clinical educator
- apply learning theories that are appropriate for adult and professional learners
- plan, implement and facilitate learning in the clinical setting
- apply sound principles and judgement in the assessment of performance in the clinical setting
- evaluate the learning experience
- reflect on experience and formulate action plans to improve future practice.

Revalidation

Revalidation demonstrates competence and maintenance of standards to the public. In some countries this is called 'maintenance of professional standards.'[15] The Federation of Medical Regulatory Authorities of Canada (FMRAC) defines revalidation as:

> A quality assurance process in which members of a . . . medical regulatory authority are required to provide satisfactory evidence of their commitment to continued competence in their practice.[16]

Formal, enforced revalidation is a relatively new concept for doctors. In 2007 the FMRAC issued a position statement which outlined that:

> All licensed physicians in Canada must participate in a recognised revalidation process in which they demonstrate their commitment to continued competent performance in a framework that is fair, relevant, inclusive, transferable and formative.[12]

Although the FMRAC had no authority to implement changes, subsequent agreement with this statement resulted in moves for appropriate policy changes to support this process.[17] Revalidation is being introduced by the General Medical Council (GMC) for doctors in the UK.[18] From 2009, UK doctors must be licensed by the GMC to practise. All licensed doctors will undergo five-yearly revalidation consisting of three elements (*see* Box 1.10). One component, recertification, has been in practice in the USA for many years.[19] The goal of recertification has been defined as being to:

> improve the quality of medical care by ensuring that the certified internist and subspecialist possess the knowledge, skills and attitudes essential to the provision of excellent care.[20]

Revalidation with the GMC will occur from 2012, and requires doctors to collect information about all of their professional work, including teaching and training, as follows:[21]
➤ appraisal – required annually within the workplace
➤ continuing professional development (CPD)/continuing medical education (CME)
➤ clinical audit
➤ patient and colleague feedback
➤ other quality measures of performance.

TABLE 1.2 Mapping professional standards to supporting information and evidence. Adapted from The Map of the RCGP's Criteria, Standards and Evidence to the GMC's Revalidation Framework[4]

GMC attribute	RCGP suggested supporting evidence and evaluation
Domain 1: knowledge, skills and performance	
Maintain your professional performance	Continuing professional development credits
	Multi-source feedback with evidence[a]
	Evaluations of teaching and appraisals by learners and appraisers
Apply knowledge and experience to practice	Patient (and/or learner) evaluations[a]
	Multi-source feedback from colleagues[a]
	Review of formal complaints[b]
Keep clear, accurate and legible records	Multi-source feedback from colleagues[a]
Domain 2: safety and quality	
Put into effect systems to protect patients and improve care	Evidence of active and effective participation in regular and sufficient appraisals
	PDP and review of last PDP, at least annually, with reflection on whether educational needs have been met
	Significant event audits[b]
	Review of formal complaints[b]
	Audits of care/practice[c]
Respond to risks to safety (or risks to unsupervised learners for whom you are responsible)	Evidence and supporting statements for training, standards of care and competence in any extended role performed
	Multi-source feedback from colleagues[a]
	Evidence of appropriate insurance/indemnity cover

GMC attribute	RCGP suggested supporting evidence and evaluation
Protect patients and colleagues from any risk posed by your health	Statement of health and use of healthcare
	Multi-source feedback from colleagues[a]
Domain 3: communication, partnership and teamwork	
Communicate effectively	Multi-source feedback from colleagues[a]
Work constructively with colleagues and delegate effectively	Multi-source feedback from colleagues[a]
Establish and maintain partnership with patients (and/or learners)	Patient (and/or learner) evaluations[a]
	Multi-source feedback from colleagues[a]
	Review of formal complaints[b]
Domain 4: maintaining trust	
Show respect for patients (and/or learners)	Patient (and/or learner) evaluations[a]
	Multi-source feedback from colleagues[a]
	Review of formal complaints[b]
Treat patients (and learners) and colleagues fairly and without discrimination	Patient (and/or learner) evaluations[a]
	Multi-source feedback from colleagues[a]
	Review of formal complaints[b]
Act with honesty and integrity	Statement of probity
	Multi-source feedback from colleagues[a]

a With evidence of appropriate reflection, change and discussion in appraisal.
b With description of circumstances, lessons learned, appropriate action taken and discussion in appraisal.
c With standards, re-audit and evidence of appropriate improvement, compliance with best-practice guidelines and discussion in appraisal.

BOX 1.10 Elements of GMC revalidation for UK doctors[18]

1 To confirm that licensed doctors practise in accordance with the GMC's generic standards (relicensing).
2 To confirm that doctors on the GMC's specialist register or GP register continue to meet the standards appropriate for their specialty (recertification).
3 To identify for further investigation, and remediation, poor practice where local systems are not robust enough to do this or do not exist.

Revalidation has been ingrained for some time among UK nurses and midwives under post-registration education and practice (PREP) requirements. It requires nurses and midwives to practise for a minimum of 450 hours per annum and to undertake at least 35 hours of CPD. They must record their learning activities and the way that these have 'informed and influenced' their practice over the three years in order to renew their professional registration, without which they cannot practise as a nurse or midwife in the UK.[22]

If practitioners are maintaining an up-to-date, comprehensive portfolio and are undertaking regular CPD and appraisal, much of the supporting information required for revalidation will already be available. Practitioners must record both what they have done and how they have implemented their learning in practice. Although formal revalidation may not currently apply to healthcare teachers, this situation may change as the need for public accountability increases. Teachers must help learners to prepare for relicensing/revalidation exercises and/or be the assessors undertaking these processes. Therefore teachers must understand the need for and the principles and processes of revalidation.

REFERENCES

1 Cate OT, Durning S. Peer teaching in medical education: twelve reasons to move from theory to practice. *Med Teach.* 2007; **29**: 591–9.
2 Mackinnon R, Haque A, Stark P. Peer teaching: by students for students. A student-led initiative. *Clin Teacher.* 2009; **6**: 245–8.
3 Nursing and Midwifery Council. *Standards for the Preparation and Practice of Supervisors of Midwives.* London: Nursing and Midwifery Council; 2006. www.nmc-uk.org
4 Royal College of General Practitioners. *RCGP Guide to the Revalidation of General Practitioners. Version 4.* London: Royal College of General Practitioners; 2010. www.rcgp.org.uk/PDF/PDS_Guide_to_Revalidation_for_GPs.pdf
5 Syder B, Kent A. *Phoenix Agenda.* Leeds: NHS Executive; 1998.
6 Garcarz W. *Primary Care Group Formation. Organisational development tools.* Birmingham: Birmingham Health Authority; 1998.
7 Roach S. *The Human Act of Caring: a blueprint for health professions.* Ottawa, ON: Canadian Hospital Association Press; 1992.
8 Benner P. *From Novice to Expert: excellence and power in clinical nursing practice.* Menlo Park, CA: Addison-Wesley; 1984.
9 Royal College of General Practitioners. *Portfolio-Based Learning in General Practice.* Occasional Paper 63. London: Royal College of General Practitioners; 1993.

10 Woodrow M. The struggle for the soul of life-long learning. *Widening Participation and Lifelong Learning.* 1999; **1:** 9–12.

11 Schreyer Institute for Teaching Excellence. *Items to Consider Including in a Teaching/ Learning Portfolio.* Penn State University; 2007. www.schreyerinstitute.psu.edu/pdf/ TandLPortfolioMaterialsToInclude.pdf

12 Mohanna K, Chambers R, Wall D. *Your Teaching Style: a practical guide to understanding, developing and improving.* Oxford: Radcliffe Publishing; 2008.

13 Academy of Medical Educators. *Professional Standards.* London: Academy of Medical Educators; 2009. www.medicaleducators.org/uploadedcontent/AoME%20 Professional%20Standards.pdf

14 Chartered Society of Physiotherapy. *Accreditation of Clinical Educators Scheme Guidance.* London: Chartered Society of Physiotherapy; 2004. www.csp.org.uk/uploads/documents/ csp_ace_scheme_guidance.pdf

15 Newble D, Paget N, McLaren B. Revalidation in Australia and New Zealand: approach of Royal Australasian College of Physicians. *BMJ.* 1999; **319:** 1185–8.

16 Federation of Medical Regulatory Authorities of Canada Revalidation Working Group. *Physician Revalidation: maintaining competence and performance.* Ottawa, ON: FMRAC; 2007. www.fmrac.ca/committees/documents/final_reval_position_eng.pdf

17 Levinson W. Revalidation of physicians in Canada: are we passing the test? *Can Med Assoc J.* 2008; **179:** 979–80.

18 General Medical Council. *Revalidation.* www.gmc-uk.org/doctors/7330.asp

19 Norcini JJ. Recertification in the United States. *BMJ.* 1999; **319:** 1183–5.

20 Benson JA. Certification and recertification: one approach to professional accountability. *Ann Intern Med.* 1991; **114:** 238–42.

21 General Medical Council. *Standards for Revalidating Doctors.* London: General Medical Council; 2010. www.gmc-uk.org/doctors/revalidation/revalidation_relicensing.asp

22 Nursing and Midwifery Council. *The PREP Handbook.* London: Nursing and Midwifery Council; 2008. www.nmc-uk.org/Educators/Standards-for-education/The-Prep-handbook/

FURTHER READING

- Baldwin S. *The Midwifery Lecturer Practitioner in Practice.* Midwives Online; 2008. www. rcm.org.uk/midwives/in-depth-papers/the-midwifery-lecturer-practitioner-in-practice

- Chambers R, Tavabie A, Mohanna K *et al.* Making the most of appraisal: when being appraised. In: *The Good Appraisal Toolkit for Primary Care.* Oxford: Radcliffe Publishing; 2004.

- Deighan M, Mohanna K. Planning learning in the new curriculum. In: *General Practice Specialty Training.* London: Royal College of General Practitioners; 2008. pp. 153–62.

- Hardicre J. Meeting the requirements for becoming a nurse lecturer. *Nurs Times.* 2003; **99:** 32–5. www.nursingtimes.net/nursing-practice-clinical-research/meeting-the-requirements -for-becoming-a-nurse-lecturer/205217.article

- Nursing and Midwifery Council. *Standards to Support Learning and Assessment in Practice.* London: Nursing and Midwifery Council; 2008. www.nmc-uk.org/Educators/ standards-for-education/standards-to-support-learning-and-assessment-in-practice/

- Schreyer Institute for Teaching Excellence. *Teaching and Course Portfolios.* www.schreyer institute.psu.edu/Tools/Portfolios

- Wilson FC. Teaching by residents. In: *Graduate Medical Education.* Oxford: Radcliffe Publishing; 2009. pp. 83–91.

CHAPTER 2

Healthcare professionals as teachers

All healthcare professionals are teachers. Daily interactions with patients, carers, staff and colleagues result in challenges to and development of knowledge, skills and beliefs. Patients expect you to explain risk and increase their understanding of diagnoses, investigations and management options. In all patient contacts you should aim to increase their understanding of their condition, in order to maximise their involvement in decision making. These are teaching skills. Multi-professional working requires you to call on the strengths of all team members, appreciate aspects of healthcare from another's perspective, gain insight into patients' needs and help everyone to remain up to date. Colleagues, who may not think of themselves as teachers, may give presentations, run sessions (e.g. journal clubs) or chair meetings and be involved in the educational setting in its widest sense.

As you undertake these tasks, you will draw on the skills of communication and active listening, which are integral to the role of healthcare providers. Learner-centredness is akin to patient-centredness, and there are many transferable skills from patient care that you can use in teaching (see Box 2.1).

FORMAL AND INFORMAL TEACHING ROLES AMONG HEALTHCARE PROFESSIONALS

Informal teaching by role modelling, observation and apprenticeship has a long and distinguished history in the perpetuation of clinical skills, professional roles and responsibilities. Teaching is an integral aspect of the healthcare provider's role. Indeed the Hippocratic Oath includes reference to teaching:

> I swear by Apollo the physician . . . to teach others this art, without fee and covenant; to give a share of precepts and oral instruction and all the other learning to those who have taken this oath under medical law.[2]

In modern times the following part of the oath is still in practice worldwide:

Through their scholarly activities, [physicians] contribute to the creation, dissemination, application and translation of medical knowledge. As teachers they facilitate the education of their students, patients, colleagues and others.[3]

BOX 2.1 Skills for good interpersonal communication
(adapted from Tate[1])

1 Listen with genuine interest.
2 Create a conducive environment.
3 Be encouraging.
4 Show understanding and empathy.
5 Check current understanding.
6 Reflect/summarise and paraphrase answers.
7 Use closed questions for exploration.
8 Use open questions for clarification.
9 Adopt a similar language and avoid jargon.
10 Use plural pronouns to indicate partnership.
11 Be provisional rather than dogmatic.
12 Be descriptive not judgemental.
13 Comment on the issues rather than on personalities.
14 Encourage eye contact.
15 Give information in clear, simple terms and use repetition.
16 Check understanding.
17 Use silence.

According to worldwide professional bodies, doctors are responsible for teaching students and colleagues (*see* Box 2.2).[4–7] Globally, all healthcare professionals are expected to take responsibility for the education of colleagues, trainees (*see* Box 2.3),[8–10] patients and the public (*see* Box 2.4).[5,11]

BOX 2.2 Responsibilities of doctors with regard to teaching
colleagues and students

UK General Medical Council, as stated in *Tomorrow's Doctors*:[4]

'Doctors are responsible for:
  a) Following the principles of professional practice that are set out in *Good Medical Practice*, including being willing to contribute to the education of students.
  b) Developing the skills and practice of a competent teacher if they are involved in teaching.
  c) Supervising the students for whom they are responsible, to support their learning and ensure patient safety.
  d) Providing objective, honest and timely assessments of the students they are asked to appraise or assess.

e) Providing feedback on students' performance.
f) Meeting contractual requirements, including any that relate to teaching.'

American Academy of Family Physicians:[5]

'All family medicine residency graduates should:
. . . facilitate continuous learning and quality improvement for all members of the healthcare team.'

Canadian Medical Association, as stated in the *CMA Code of Ethics:*[6]

'Be willing to teach and learn from medical students, other colleagues and other health professionals.'

Australian Medical Association, as stated in the *Code of Ethics:*[7]

'Honour your obligation to pass on your professional knowledge and skills to colleagues and students [and] refrain from exploiting students or colleagues under your supervision in any way.'

BOX 2.3 Responsibilities of non-medical healthcare professionals with regard to teaching colleagues and students

UK Nursing and Midwifery Council, as stated in *The Code: standards of conduct, performance and ethics for nurses and midwives:*[8]

'You must be willing to share your skills and experience for the benefit of your colleagues.'

Canadian Nurses Association, as stated in the *Code of Ethics for Registered Nurses:*[9]

'Nurses share their knowledge and provide feedback, mentorship and guidance for the professional development of nursing students, novice nurses and other health-care team members.'

UK College of Occupational Therapists, as stated in the *Code of Ethics and Professional Conduct:*[10]

'You have a professional responsibility to provide regular practice education opportunities for occupational therapy students where possible, and to promote a learning culture within the workplace.'

BOX 2.4 Responsibilities of all healthcare professionals with regard to teaching patients and the public

American Academy of Family Physicians:[5]

'Family physicians should take a leadership role in improving the health of the American public by providing accurate and meaningful patient education.'

World Medical Association, as stated in the *International Code of Medical Ethics*[11]

'A physician shall recognise his/her important role in educating the public but should use due caution in divulging discoveries or new techniques or treatment through non-professional channels.'

Traditionally (in the education of juniors), formal healthcare teaching qualifications or roles were not the norm. Clinical teachers may have ended up in that post as a result of their seniority and clinical experience, rather than by training and educational experience. Teachers in higher education may enter their roles as a result of their research experience. For example, hospital consultants frequently act as educational supervisors of junior doctors, with little or no formal training in that role.

However, nurses, general practitioners and therapists have established more rigorous approaches to the preparation of teachers. The buddy or assistant-operator pairing is a much more formal version of the 'sitting with Nelly' observational form of teaching, and is used in the training and assessment of dentists.

Both formal and informal, recognised and unrecognised teaching roles exist within healthcare, and the need and opportunity for such roles are increasing. The role of the healthcare professional as teacher is 'a core professional activity that cannot be left to chance, aptitude or inclination.'[12]

Increasingly, educational roles are expected of nurses and midwives, and are part of their contract of employment. In these formal roles, a distinction is drawn between mentors, assessors, practice educators and lecturers.[13] Slightly different competences are expected within these different roles. These definitions (*see* Box 2.5) are primarily for nursing, midwifery and health visiting, but the competences defined can be generalised to other health professions.

BOX 2.5 Teaching role definitions of the English National Board for Nursing, Midwifery and Health Visiting[13]

- The term 'mentor' denotes the role of the nurse, midwife or health visitor who facilitates learning and supervises and assesses students in the practice setting. In nursing, the term 'assessor' is often used to denote a role similar to that of the mentor.
- The term 'practice educator' denotes the role of the teacher of nursing, midwifery or health visiting, who:
  - makes a significant contribution to education in the practice setting, coordinating student experiences and assessment of learning

- leads the development of practice
- provides support and guidance to mentors and others who contribute to the students' experience in practice, enabling students to meet learning outcomes and develop appropriate competencies.
- The term 'lecturer' denotes the role of the teacher of nursing, midwifery or health visiting employed in an educational institution, who has responsibility for the development and delivery of educational programmes in nursing, midwifery or health visiting.

Please note that the definitions are different for other healthcare disciplines (*see* Chapter 18).

The UK Nursing and Midwifery Council (NMC) advisory standards for nursing mentors are listed in Box 2.6.[14]

BOX 2.6 UK Nursing and Midwifery Council (NMC) advisory standards for nursing mentors[14]

Effective [nursing] mentors will develop:
- Communication and working relationships that enable:
  - the development of effective relationships based on mutual trust and respect
  - an understanding of how learners integrate into practice settings, and assist with this process
  - the provision of ongoing and constructive support for learners.
- Facilitation of learning in order to:
  - demonstrate sufficient knowledge of the learner's programme to identify current learning needs
  - demonstrate strategies that will assist with the integration of learning from practice and educational settings
  - create and develop opportunities for learners to identify and undertake experiences to meet their learning needs.
- Assessment in order to:
  - demonstrate a good understanding of assessment and ability to assess
  - implement approved assessment procedures.
- Role modelling in order to:
  - demonstrate effective relationships with patients and clients
  - contribute to the development of an environment in which effective practice is fostered, implemented, evaluated and disseminated
  - assess and manage clinical developments to ensure safe and effective care.
- Creation of an environment for learning in order to:
  - ensure effective learning experiences and the opportunity to achieve learning outcomes for students by contributing to the development and maintenance of a learning environment
  - implement strategies for quality assurance and quality audit.
- Improvement of practice in order to:

- contribute to the creation of an environment in which change can be initiated and supported.
- A knowledge base in order to:
  - identify, apply and disseminate research findings within the area of practice.
- Course development which:
  - contributes to the development and/or review of courses.

Please note that the definition of mentor for UK nurses is different to that for other healthcare disciplines (*see* Chapter 18).

RESPONDING TO CHANGING HEALTHCARE SYSTEMS AND EDUCATIONAL INFRASTRUCTURES

The impact of continuing changes in and modernisation of healthcare systems is felt in training and education through changes in patient care patterns and working arrangements. For example, there is recognition of the detrimental effect on high-quality graduate medical education of the long hours worked, reduced length of inpatient stays and the 'increased acuity of the average inpatient' that place additional demands on juniors' time and energy.[15] In 2004, the introduction of the European Working Time Directive (EWTD) aimed to improve the work–life balance of UK doctors, and subsequently improve patient care. However, this has resulted in less time being available for teaching and training, due to a direct reduction in clinical exposure and changes to rotas, with subsequent staff shortages. More frequent handovers and reduced exposure to each patient prevent follow-up throughout a patient's admission, and this risks training jobs becoming focused on service provision rather than training. Calls to formalise training and define the competences of educational supervisors of UK junior doctors are being addressed.[16] 'An international trend across all healthcare sectors towards formalising the role and training of work-based educators' has been identified.[16]

A review of the UK postgraduate medical education and training system[17] recognised an 'erosion' of the 'traditional clinical academic departments' and the existence of fewer clinical academic posts in medical schools, resulting in increased reliance on clinical staff to deliver undergraduate teaching and postgraduate supervision. Integrated educational and clinical training pathways were suggested to facilitate formal training, development and qualification in educational skills.[17]

A significant problem in the USA is faculty shortages at nursing schools due to budget constraints that have made salaries for teachers lower compared with those for clinical or private-sector workers. Furthermore, the ageing population of faculty staff will soon result in a wave of faculty retirements.[18] Multiple initiatives have been introduced to improve funding for individuals who are entering a career in education, and to provide funding for increased numbers of faculty staff in schools of nursing.[18]

Funding for education is dynamic and vulnerable due to changing healthcare system and political priorities. Funding overhauls can either be beneficial or detrimental to various groups of healthcare professionals at different levels, particularly if disparities among groups are recognised. Significant changes can be implemented at relatively short notice.[19] Therefore teachers must be equipped, adequately represented and supported to provide good-quality education in a flexible and changing environment.

The landscape in which medical education and training is taking place is changing, and a number of different organisations have a role in shaping the environment in ways which affect doctors' careers and learning. The challenge for the regulator is to maintain standards within a framework that is robust but flexible enough to be applied regardless of the organisation changes that might take place within the . . . healthcare system.'[20]

RECOGNISING THE NEED FOR HIGH-QUALITY TEACHING STAFF

There must be an adequate supply of high-quality teaching staff in both academic and clinical settings. Healthcare professionals should be taught by those with recent practical experience. The availability of flexible multi-professional education and training for all healthcare professions has been a crucial initial development.[21] In the USA, this need is being addressed by the development of ten recommendations that integrate core competences into the education of healthcare professionals to create reform by enhancing quality and meeting the changing needs and demands of patients.[22] The goal of developing high-quality teaching staff has been further reinforced by an emphasis on continuing professional development/continuous medical education, lifelong learning, increasing training commissions for healthcare professionals, inter-professional learning and working, and preparing students and staff for new roles and new ways of working.[23] In the UK, formalisation of these values[17] has resulted in the development of a single organisation (Medical Education England), which aims to provide professional leadership of workforce planning and education for medical staff. This should be followed by the development of similar bodies for other healthcare professionals.

With the goal of developing high-quality teaching staff, it becomes necessary to formally define the role and skills of an effective teacher in the healthcare professions.

DEFINING AN EFFECTIVE TEACHER

The roles, qualities and skills of a healthcare professional who is a competent teacher have been described elsewhere.[24] Healthcare professionals who are formally appointed to provide clinical or educational supervision of those in training, or who undertake to provide training or supervision for students, should demonstrate the following personal and professional attributes:

➤ commitment to the appropriate professional guidance (e.g. *Good Medical Practice*[24])
➤ enthusiasm for their specialty
➤ personal commitment to teaching and learning
➤ sensitivity and responsiveness to the educational needs of learners
➤ the capacity to promote development of the required professional attitudes and values
➤ understanding of the principles of education as applied to healthcare
➤ understanding of research methods
➤ practical teaching skills
➤ willingness to develop both as a healthcare professional and as a teacher
➤ commitment to audit and peer review of their teaching
➤ the ability to use formative assessment for the benefit of the learner
➤ the ability to carry out formal appraisal of students' progress and/or the performance of the trainee as a practising professional.

The core content of the clinical teaching role was identified by asking consultants and junior hospital doctors what they thought the curriculum should be for teaching medical teachers.[25] Harden and Crosby have also published the roles of a medical teacher.[26]

DEFINING EXCELLENCE AMONG TEACHERS

A framework for developing excellence as a clinical educator[27] categorises activity into performance of tasks ('doing the right thing'), approach to tasks ('doing the thing right') and professionalism ('the right person doing it'). Sometimes we can only define good teaching as what a good teacher does.[12] Context and application have much to do with the standards to which we aspire.

The criteria set out within *Good Medical Practice for General Practitioners*[28] (*see* Box 2.7) describe the excellent teacher, the definition of 'excellence' being 'meets the "exemplary GP" criteria all or nearly all of the time.'

BOX 2.7 Criteria for the exemplary GP teacher[28]

In addition to the attributes of an effective teacher, the criteria for the exemplary GP teacher include the following:

- Ensures that patients are not put at risk when seeing students or doctors in training.
- Offers the patient an open opportunity, without pressure, to decide whether to take part in a teaching consultation.
- Uses formative assessment and constructs educational plans.
- Assists in making honest assessments of learners.

In the UK, *Professional Standards for Medical Educators*[29] outline the expectations of these professionals. All teachers can compare their practice against these standards to assess their performance level and to identify areas for development.

CONCLUSION

In order to meet organisational and other changes within the healthcare system it is increasingly important to formalise teaching. Many varied ways of defining a healthcare teacher's role and how well they perform are being developed. Important changes are also occurring in the way that teaching is delivered in formal settings.

However, all healthcare professionals teach at some time. Efficient use of teaching time includes harnessing the potential for informal contacts to enhance learning. The Conference of Postgraduate Medical Deans (CoPMeD)[30] proposed the following model, which describes the potential in every contact between trainee and trainer.[31]

Learning from the current patient or clinical opportunity	Building on previous learning experience
Opportunistic education, training and learning	Modification of learning behaviour

---

Tips from experienced teachers

When branching into teaching from your core job as a healthcare professional, value your 'transferable skills':

- creating rapport with patients (or with learners)
- listening to patients (or learners, hearing their learning needs)
- giving information in ways that patients (or learners) understand and that answer their questions (i.e. giving it at the right level and at the right time).

REFERENCES

1 Tate P. *The Doctor's Communication Handbook*. 3rd edn. Oxford: Radcliffe Medical Press; 2000.

2 Beauchamp T, Walters L. The Hippocratic Oath. In: *Contemporary Issues in Bioethics*. Encino, CA: Dickenson; 1978.

3 Frank JR, ed. *The CanMEDS 2005 Physician Competency Framework*. Ottawa, ON: Royal College of Physicians and Surgeons of Canada; 2005. http://rcpsc.medical.org/canmeds/CanMEDS2005/CanMEDS2005_e.pdf

4 General Medical Council. *Tomorrow's Doctors*. London: General Medical Council; 2009. www.gmc-uk.org/static/documents/content/TomorrowsDoctors_2009.pdf

5 American Academy of Family Physicians. *Expectations of Family Medicine Residency Graduates*. www.aafp.org/online/en/home/policy/policies/e/expoffmrgrads.html

6 Canadian Medical Association. *CMA Code of Ethics*. Ottawa, ON: Canadian Medical Association; 2004. http://policybase.cma.ca/PolicyPDF/PD04-06.pdf

7 Australian Medical Association. *Code of Ethics*. Kingston, ACT: Australian Medical Association; 2006. www.ama.com.au/codeofethics

8 Nursing and Midwifery Council. *The Code: standards of conduct, performance and ethics for nurses and midwives*. London: Nursing and Midwifery Council; 2008. www.nmc-uk.org/aDisplayDocument.aspx?documentID=5982

9 Canadian Nurses Association. *Code of Ethics for Registered Nurses*. Ottawa, ON: Canadian Nurses Association; 2008. www.cna-nurses.ca/CNA/documents/pdf/publications/Code_of_Ethics_2008_e.pdf

10 College of Occupational Therapists. *Code of Ethics and Professional Conduct*. Revised edn. London: College of Occupational Therapists; 2010. www.cot.co.uk/Mainwebsite/Resources/Document/Code-of-Ethics_2010.pdf

11 World Medical Association. *International Code of Medical Ethics*. 2006. www.wma.net/en/30publications/10policies/c8/index.html

12 Purcell N, Lloyd-Jones G. Standards for medical educators. *Med Educ*. 2003; **37**: 149–54.

13 English National Board for Nursing, Midwifery and Health Visiting and Department of Health. *Preparation of Mentors and Teachers*. London: English National Board and Department of Health; 2001.

14 Nursing and Midwifery Council. *Standards for the Preparation of Teachers of Nursing and Midwifery*. London: Nursing and Midwifery Council; 2002.

15 Association of American Medical Colleges. *AAMC Policy Guidance on Graduate Medical Education: assuring quality patient care and quality education*. Washington, DC: Association of American Medical Colleges; 2001. www.aamc.org/patientcare/gmepolicy/gmepolicy.pdf

16 Academy of Medical Educators. *Educational Supervisors in Secondary Care. Stage 1 report. Executive summary.* London: Academy of Medical Educators; 2009. www.nact.org.uk/pdf_documents/Education%20Supervisor%20Stage%201%20Summary.pdf

17 Tooke J. *Aspiring to Excellence: findings and final recommendations of the Independent Inquiry into Modernising Medical Careers.* London: MMC Inquiry; 2008.

18 American Association of Colleges of Nursing. *Nursing Faculty Shortage Fact Sheet.* Washington, DC: American Association of Colleges of Nursing; 2010. www.aacn.nche.edu/Media/FactSheets/NursingShortage.htm

19 Next Stage Review Implementation Team. *High Quality Care For All: our journey so far.* London: Department of Health; 2009.

20 General Medical Council and the Postgraduate Medical Education and Training Board. *Report of the Education and Training Regulation Policy Review: recommendations and options for the future regulation of education and training.* London: General Medical Council; 2010. https://gmc.e-consultation.net/econsult/uploaddocs/Consult115/Patel%20Review%20Report.pdf

21 Department of Health. *A Health Service of All the Talents: developing the NHS workforce.* London: Department of Health; 2000.

22 Greiner AC, Knebel E, Committee on the Health Professions Education Summit. *Health Professions Education: a bridge to quality.* Washington, DC: The National Academies Press; 2003. www.acme-assn.org/valuable_resources/IOM-ABridgetoQuality.pdf

23 Department of Health. *The NHS Plan: a plan for investment, a plan for reform.* London: Department of Health; 2000.

24 General Medical Council. *Good Medical Practice.* London: General Medical Council; 2006. www.gmc-uk.org/static/documents/content/GMC_0510.pdf

25 Wall D, McAleer S. Teaching the consultant teachers: identifying the core content. *Med Educ.* 2000; **34**: 131–8.

26 Harden R, Crosby JR. *The Good Teacher is More Than a Lecturer: the twelve roles of the teacher.* AMEE Education Guide 20. Dundee: Centre for Medical Education; 2000.

27 Hesketh EA, Bagnall G, Buckley EG *et al.* A framework for developing excellence as a clinical educator. *Med Educ.* 2001; **35**: 555–64.

28 Royal College of General Practitioners, General Practitioners Committee. *Good Medical Practice for General Practitioners.* London: Royal College of General Practitioners; 2008.

29 Academy of Medical Educators. *Professional Standards for Medical Educators.* London: Academy of Medical Educators; 2009. www.medicaleducators.org/uploadedcontent/AoME%20Professional%20Standards.pdf

30 Department of Health. *European Working Time Directive.* www.doh.gov.uk

31 Conference of Postgraduate Medical Deans (CoPMeD). *Liberating Learning: a practical guide for learners and teachers to postgraduate medical education and the European Working Time Directive.* London: Conference of Postgraduate Medical Deans; 2002.

FURTHER READING

• Association of Faculties of Medicine of Canada. *The Future of Medical Education in Canada (FMEC): a collective vision for MD education.* Ottawa, ON: Association of Faculties of Medicine of Canada; 2010. www.afmc.ca/fmec/pdf/collective_vision.pdf

• Wilson FC. Work hours and the supervision of residents. In: *Graduate Medical Education.* Oxford: Radcliffe Publishing; 2009. pp. 49–55.

CHAPTER 3

Healthcare teaching in context

Healthcare systems and education are closely linked. A change in one will inevitably bring about (the need for) change in the other. Significant events or inquiries into healthcare systems can initiate change within both clinical and educational structures. For example, the Bristol Royal Infirmary Inquiry into avoidable deaths of children recommended prioritising the following non-clinical aspects of care in education, training and continuing professional development (CPD) of health professionals:[1]

➤ skills in communicating with patients and with colleagues
➤ education about the principles and organisation of the healthcare service, about how care is managed, and the skills required for management
➤ development of teamwork
➤ shared learning across professional boundaries
➤ clinical audit and reflective practice (*see* Chapter 5)
➤ leadership (*see* Chapter 19).

This chapter demonstrates how changing healthcare services changes learning needs, and how these needs can be met through inter-professional learning, CPD and the development of appropriate education and training programmes. Other important related concepts include evidence-based education (*see* Chapter 21) and reviewing your own performance (*see* Chapter 1).

CHANGING HEALTHCARE SERVICES CHANGES LEARNING NEEDS

Changes in the focus of healthcare delivery create new educational and training needs for healthcare professionals, managers and other non-clinical staff. For example, changes in the UK healthcare services[2] resulted in learning needs centred around commissioning and delivery of healthcare that is better informed by local issues, and targeting of services more directly at local health needs to reduce inequalities. Basing clinical care, management or health policy on evidence, when available, or being able to justify performance where it diverts from the norm or best practice, continue to be learning needs for many healthcare professionals. These complex areas require as great an understanding of the context of the topics as the subject areas themselves. For instance, changing approaches to developing healthcare services involves learning more about 'health needs assessment', and requires knowledge about the differences and interrelationships between 'need' (the potential to benefit from care), 'demand' (expressed desire for services) and 'supply' (services that are actually provided in relation to need or demand). Public health has adopted a population-based perspective, whereas clinicians traditionally focus on the needs of individual patients. Now, healthcare workers and managers must take a 'macro' *and* 'micro' perspective on 'health', rather than just considering individual patients. They must also develop the skills to manage the conflict that results from using both approaches. The educational requirements and learning needs of people working in healthcare services are diverse (*see* Box 3.1).

BOX 3.1 Educational requirements of today's healthcare services

- Education and training plans should complement those of the individual unit or practice, healthcare organisations and central priorities.
- Implementation of clinical governance, quality assurance and safety measures: knowledge, positive attitudes, new skills and learning culture.
- Adoption of evidence-based practice: where and how to get information, how to apply evidence and monitor changes.
- Needs assessments: how to conduct them, who to work with, linking needs assessment with commissioning and providing care, finding ways to reduce health inequalities.
- Working in partnerships: with other disciplines, clinicians and managers, clinicians and patients or the public, others from non-health organisations.
- Involving the public and patients in planning and delivering healthcare.
- Health service management developments: understanding and working with new models of delivery of care; as work-based teams and across primary/secondary care interfaces.
- Delivering tangible outcomes: thinking and planning in terms of 'health gains' rather than improvements in structures and systems.
- Research and development: encouraging a culture whereby the two are inextricably linked; healthcare professionals having critical appraisal skills.

Acceptance and application of patient and public involvement in decision making requires healthcare professionals to develop new attitudes and beliefs, and not just to update their knowledge and skills. Such cultural changes will only be achieved if traditional boundaries between healthcare professionals and patients, or between the healthcare service and the voluntary sector, are eradicated. Achieving quality improvements and establishing a clinical governance culture requires everyone's willing cooperation. Healthcare professionals, managers and patients need to develop a responsibility, and learn the skills necessary, for delivering cost-effective, evidence-based, acceptable, safe and successful care.

Focusing education on the needs of the learner and healthcare system

Education must be focused and relevant to the needs of the learner, patients *and* the healthcare system.[3,4] The traditional approach to education has been to segregate the professions and to allow individuals to opt for postgraduate courses based on personal preferences rather than service needs. This is no longer tenable. Inter-professional and needs-based training is now essential if the healthcare workforce is to have 'the capacity, skills, diversity and flexibility to meet the demands on the service' that are now envisaged as being integral to the delivery of modern healthcare services.[5]

Common priorities for education and training from local, district and national perspectives can overlap. Education and training needs should be assessed against all of these development priorities so that educational programmes are relevant to service needs.

Ever changing educational and training needs cannot be met by sending individuals on various ad-hoc courses. Service changes affect everyone, so a coordinated approach to educational provision is needed at local levels if the healthcare service is to deliver new models of care that better target the needs of the community.

Teachers should support individual learners to follow programmes of activities that are matched to their own predetermined educational plans. They should also help individuals to design plans to complement the overall business and development plans of their local healthcare service to deliver central and district priorities.

Teachers are crucial in helping learners to identify the modes of education delivery that are best suited to their planned activities. A survey of the education and training needs of primary care professionals showed how professionals from ten different disciplines tended to opt for the mode of training with which they were most familiar (usually a lecture or a validated professional course) or which suited their working conditions (e.g. distance learning for those who found it difficult to take study leave from their workplace). Few matched their educational requirements with the mode of delivery that was most appropriate for the topic.[6]

You may need to acquire new knowledge and skills to become more aware of, and expert in, reconciling the needs of individual healthcare professionals and organisations, or recommendations from external sources such as providers of national guidelines and service frameworks. The learning culture for the modern healthcare systems cannot be delivered simply through lectures or seminars, but requires a partnership between educationalists, managers and healthcare professionals, and imaginative educational programmes.

INTER-PROFESSIONAL EDUCATION

Quality care usually results from effective multi-professional partnerships. Working in partnerships with a wide range of healthcare disciplines requires learning about the roles, responsibilities and capabilities of other professionals. Inter-professional education has been internationally advocated to improve the way that multi-professional teams work together:

> All health professionals should be educated to deliver patient-centred care as members of an interdisciplinary team, emphasizing evidence-based practice, quality improvement approaches, and informatics.[7]

A widely cited definition of inter-professional education is:

> when two or more professions learn with, from and about each other to improve collaboration and the quality of care.[8]

Others describe multi-professional education as:

> when members of two or more professions simply learn side by side whatever the purpose.[9]

Thus inter-professional education involves the participation of, communication and interaction between, and active listening among learners of different professions – not just a roomful of learners silently listening to a lecture.[9,10]

Benefits of inter-professional education

The benefits of inter-professional education include:[9,11–14]
➤ reduced isolation of different professionals
➤ enhancement of the collaborative approach necessary for cost-effective delivery of quality and safe care and for meeting the needs of local communities, including the development of competences in:[15]
  — group decision making
  — teamwork
  — leadership
  — conflict resolution
➤ increasing learners' understanding of others' roles and responsibilities, skills and knowledge, powers and duties, value systems and codes of conduct, opportunities and constraints[8]
➤ developing a more appropriate skill-mix of healthcare professionals, resulting in more efficient and effective employment
➤ improving patient and healthcare professional satisfaction
➤ improved access to healthcare.

A systematic review[9] looked at the evidence for inter-professional learning, and concluded that the proposed benefits listed above appear to be true, and that inter-professional learning:
➤ is generally well received, but is not accepted consistently by all learners from similar professional backgrounds
➤ is reliant on teachers being adequately competent and confident as facilitators in this setting
➤ has the potential to worsen perceptions and attitudes towards other professional groups among some learners. This must be sought, monitored and addressed by teachers.

The proposed mechanisms through which the benefits of inter-professional working and learning may occur are outlined in Box 3.2.[11]

BOX 3.2 Benefits of inter-professional working and learning[11]

The mechanisms whereby these benefits may occur include:
• development of new roles
• respect for other professions
• professionals working together in an atmosphere of openness and trust

- real communication between professionals
- an appreciation of the strengths of the diversity of other professionals and the complex nature of professional judgement and ways of working
- a common set of values and attitudes
- an understanding of the contribution that other professionals can make and how different professions work best together.

Potential barriers to inter-professional education

Inter-professional education is not always appropriate. Some subjects are so specialised that they apply to only one particular discipline or subspecialty. Participants from one discipline may not be comfortable being taught alongside other learners from a traditionally more dominant discipline, or where their learning needs are more basic than those of participants from other disciplines. This challenges inter-professional learning, where all learners should feel equal, regardless of their workplace status.[8] The evidence suggests that undergraduate inter-professional learning may not be as well received as such learning delivered at the postgraduate level,[14] perhaps because learners do not appreciate the relevance of inter-professional learning if they have yet to work in a multi-professional environment.

Practical barriers include inequalities in study budgets and study leave arrangements between professions, and different working arrangements. These differences may prevent certain groups from attending education or training events, or they may alter the perceived priority of such events. Issues such as space within learning environments may prevent or limit participation.[9]

Inter-professional education can be invaluable. However, the benefits are dependent upon the topic being taught. It appears most useful for professionals to learn about the roles of other disciplines, and least useful for them to learn about knowledge or content, as different healthcare professionals have different priorities, training and knowledge bases.

TEACHING ABOUT WORKING IN PARTNERSHIPS[16] IN THE HEALTHCARE SYSTEM

People are more likely to learn about the benefits of working in partnerships and develop new and meaningful partnerships by observing successful role models. Teaching should focus on encouraging a common understanding of people's roles, responsibilities and capabilities.

You can help people to understand more about how they perform in a certain role within a team by using psychometric or psychological measurements or interpersonal assessment, such as the Belbin Self-Perception Inventory.[17] Teams consist of individuals, with each member fulfilling a different role. Different situations dictate the role that an individual will adopt. Roles may be duplicated, or one person may play a combination of roles. All roles will be evident in any effective social or work group, although groups may survive and achieve some of their objectives with one or more of the roles unfilled.

A survey of the education and training needs of healthcare professionals and managers identified addressing the absence of effective teamwork in practices and healthcare organisations as one of their key education and training needs.[6]

The eight roles within a 'winning team' are as follows:[17]
1 chairman or coordinator: coordinates leadership, clarifies goals and priorities
2 plant: generator of ideas, solves difficult problems
3 monitor or evaluator: 'sifts' ideas, sees all the options, analyses, judges the likely outcomes
4 team worker: looks after internal relationships, listens, handles difficult people
5 resource investigator: looks after external relationships, engages in networking, explores new possibilities
6 company worker: loyal to the group, organises, turns ideas and plans into practical forms of action
7 shaper: challenges, pressurises, finds ways round obstacles
8 completer finisher: ensures that tasks and projects are completed, keeps others to schedules and targets.

The move to establish integrated team models of delivery requires more understanding of the capabilities and range of skills of the different disciplines participating, rather than just team roles.

Listed below are the positive features of partnerships that are most likely to be successful. Good partnerships between different disciplines within the healthcare system, the voluntary sector and social care depend on creating trust, mutual respect and joint working for common goals.

Tips on establishing successful working partnerships[16]

Make sure that you establish:
- a written memorandum of partnership
- a joint strategy with agreed goals and outcomes
- widespread support from individuals working within the partnership and their organisations
- clear roles and responsibilities with regard to joint working
- shared decision making on partnership matters
- that each partner has different attributes that fit well with the other partner
- partnership benefits for all organisations
- a partnership where the whole is greater than the sum of the components
- an environment where each partner makes a 'fair' investment in the partnership – and the risk–benefit balance is fair between partners
- partners who trust each other and are honest about partnership matters
- partners who appreciate, respect and tolerate each others' differences
- a common understanding about language and communication.

Teaching how to work in partnerships
➤ Set a task that requires the learner to work in partnership with others, and then analyse how that partnership was created and sustained.
➤ Encourage inter-professional learning to promote understanding of others' roles and responsibilities while undertaking an educational event.
➤ Ask the learner to gather information that is only available within other sectors,

including both healthcare settings and non-healthcare settings (e.g. housing or transport).

➤ Write case vignettes that describe situations which cross healthcare sectors and settings and involve several health disciplines. By debating who will do what, when and how, the participants will gain further understanding of other colleagues' capabilities and expertise. You might meet regularly while putting such a model into practice to address obstacles and to promote sustained changes.

CONTINUING PROFESSIONAL DEVELOPMENT (CPD)

CPD or continuing medical education (CME) has been defined as:

> a process of lifelong learning for all individuals and teams which enables professionals to expand and fulfil their potential and which also meets the needs of patients and delivers the health and healthcare priorities of the [healthcare service].[3]

The principles of CPD apply to both clinical and non-clinical staff. CPD is viewed as key to professionals' ongoing education and development, following recognition of the need to improve the quality of healthcare[18] through the processes of revalidation (*see* Chapter 1), and due to the need for greater accountability of professional competence to the public.

CPD includes:[12,18]

➤ pursuing personal and professional growth by widening, developing and changing your own roles and responsibilities

➤ keeping abreast of, and accommodating, clinical, organisational and social changes that affect professional roles in general

➤ acquiring and refining the knowledge and skills that are needed for new or current roles or responsibilities or career development

➤ putting individual development and learning needs into a team, organisational and multi-professional context.

Box 3.3[18–20] highlights the criteria for successful CPD learning. The minimum amount of CPD that should be undertaken is often defined by an individual's professional organisation. This can be increased if additional roles are taken on. For example, a UK supervisor of midwives is expected to undertake 35 hours of CPD every three years in order to renew their registration. However, they must also undertake at least 6 more hours each year to meet the standards for their educational/training role.[21]

To make the most of CPD activities you must reflect on what you have learned (*see* Chapter 5). This should usually be formally written down for your portfolio. However, in reality the process of reflection also arises through formal and informal discussions with colleagues. Evidence of attendance and the CPD 'value' of the event are often required in a portfolio, so ensure that you collect a certificate of attendance and/or accreditation whenever these are offered.

BOX 3.3 Criteria for successful CPD learning[18-20]

The most successful CPD involves learning which:
- has a clear need or reason for the particular CPD to be undertaken
- is led by the learner's own identified needs (see below, and also see Reviewing Performance in Chapter 1)
- is based on what is already known by the learner
- appropriately uses a variety of learning modalities
- involves active participation by the learner
- uses the learner's own resources
- includes relevant and timely feedback
- includes follow-up to reinforce learning (e.g. self-assessment, reflection).

Note: you should make any education or training relevant to the service needs of your healthcare system, while remembering to build on the criteria for the individual's successful learning.

LIFELONG LEARNING

Lifelong learning is a broadly based and continuous process of learning. It combines formal and informal learning, and is a natural part of everyday life.[22] Trends towards the development of a national credit framework in higher education, the accreditation of prior learning and experiential learning, the focus on learning outcomes (learners) rather than inputs (teachers), and the recognition of work and work experience as key sources of learning have all contributed to a lifelong learning culture.[23] Strong links between theory (the teaching), practice and health policy should ensure that lifelong learning applied to the healthcare services is focused on relevant service needs.[24]

BARRIERS TO TAKING UP APPROPRIATE EDUCATION

Teachers should be sufficiently flexible to cater for learners with constraints that limit their access to education, such as time, dependents, limited funds and geographical distance.[25] In addition to barriers to inter-professional learning (addressed above), Box 3.4 outlines blocks and barriers to establishing a coherent education and training programme across a practice or healthcare organisation.[26]

BOX 3.4 Blocks and barriers[26] to establishing a coherent education and training programme across a practice, unit or trust

- Isolation of healthcare professionals, even many who appear to work in a team.
- 'Tribalism' as different disciplines protect their traditional roles and responsibilities.
- Lack of incentives to take up learner-centred, interactive education as opposed to more passive modes of educational delivery.
- Various employed/attached/self-employed terms and conditions between staff employed in the same workplace, including differing rights to time and funds for continuing education.
- Lack of communication between healthcare organisations and individuals.

- Domination of the medical model over those of other disciplines.
- Rigid educational budgets of different professionals obstructing true multi-disciplinary education.
- Lack of personal educational needs assessments, which means that education may not be targeted appropriately for individual or organisational needs.
- Practitioners being overwhelmed with service work, and therefore having little time for continuing education.
- Dissonance between individuals' perceived educational needs and service relevant needs.
- Lack of shared ownership of both education and development.
- The perception that all education should be paid for by someone else.
- Conservatism – reluctance to develop or accept new models of working and extended roles.
- Selection of educational activities according to preference rather than need.
- Mental ill health – depression, stress, burnout of learner or teacher, fear of and resistance to change.

EDUCATIONAL NEEDS ASSESSMENT AND PLANNING NEW EDUCATIONAL AND TRAINING PROGRAMMES

A vast range and depth of education and training needs exist among those working in primary care,[27] and the same is likely to be true of all healthcare sectors. These needs include the following:[28]

➤ creating a healthcare organisation
➤ teamworking
➤ networking
➤ planning and management
➤ public health.

There is sometimes confusion about the differences between the terms 'education' and 'training.' Many areas of education and training bring together both functions within a learning experience. The two may be differentiated by thinking of education as being about *doing things better*, whereas training is about *taking on new tasks*.

Educational needs assessment

Educational needs assessment tools have been developed to help those in primary care to identify their learning needs.[29-31] One of these describes 29 functions and 43 skills that are needed to carry out the functions of healthcare organisations, which can be used as a comprehensive checklist to determine skill gaps and training needs.[29] Another is an organisational development tool with a skills grid based on common issues and the knowledge and personal attributes required from organisational, general management and team or practice perspectives.[30] The outcome should be to develop a learning culture while addressing those needs.[31]

Approaches to the development of new education and training programmes

The starting point for education and training programmes of many organisations is a poorly coordinated base of education and training – by individual practitioners themselves, across disciplines, between clinical and administrative staff, and between primary/community/secondary care settings. At practice or directorate level there may have been little strategic planning of the education and training needs of *all* staff, and if there has been some such planning at district or regional levels, those on the ground may not be aware of it.

Locality coordination of education and training should be arranged to ensure that programmes are networked into a district and sub-regional overview of the whole healthcare workforce. This should help to reduce duplication of resources and tailor educational provision to that needed to equip the workforce to be the most effective that the locality can afford.

When reorganising workforce training (*see* Box 3.5[32]), learning environments should be:
➤ suitable and offer opportunities to facilitate multi-disciplinary learning
➤ available in sufficient numbers to meet the training needs of the service
➤ managed, supervised and assessed by appropriately experienced and qualified professional staff
➤ quality assured and responsive to learner evaluation and feedback.

BOX 3.5 Reorganisation of workforce training[32]

1 The healthcare organisation must be clear about service needs, and about the skills and staff required to deliver those services efficiently and effectively.
2 Workforce and resources should be considered together to ensure that plans and developments are consistent and coordinated.
3 There should be an appropriate mix between central (top-down) and local (bottom-up) planning.
4 Planning should cover the whole healthcare workforce, looking across sectors (primary, secondary and tertiary), employers (public, private and voluntary) and staff groups (nurses, doctors, dentists, other professions and other staff), and should take account of evolving roles.
5 Workforce planning arrangements should reflect clear and agreed responsibilities and accountabilities, with effective performance management systems.

All healthcare organisations should appoint an education and training, professional development and workforce planning lead, to ensure that the above recommendations are met.[19]

Learning across the healthcare system should encompass the concept of lifelong learning and foster links between education, organisational development and human resources. Six themes emerging for education and training within a healthcare system are about developing a better understanding of:
➤ the nature and implementation of healthcare system changes among all staff
➤ the organisation and funding of health-related education and workforce planning systems
➤ practical links between educational providers and healthcare providers to support staff
➤ the educational and development needs of healthcare providers

➤ the development of a population focus in healthcare providers by clinicians and managers
➤ access and use of information to support learning.

Planning an appropriate education and training programme

Figure 3.1 illustrates the framework of a plan to shape an appropriate education and training programme for clinical and non-clinical healthcare staff, to meet the requirements of the healthcare system, the workforce and the local context. Start at the bottom of the page and work upwards, thinking about what the stages involve from the point of view of a healthcare provider director, manager and/or teacher:

1 Your starting point in terms of the budget, the numbers of staff, their skill base, and the extent and quality of education, training courses and activities available.
2 Preliminary identification of the education and training needs of the workforce that you are planning for. Take account of the gaps in the baseline resources that you identified, the short- and longer-term visions of development for your organisation, and how the national, district and local workforce planning strategies will affect you. Anticipate workforce trends, as there will be a lag phase of several years to recruit and train new staff.
3 Budget constraints will influence your education and training programme, as your preferred vision becomes your affordable vision. Other limitations that will influence the design of the education and training programme include the workforce's willingness to cooperate with the programme, and the need to make the programme relevant to service needs, other priorities and local issues. The design will be influenced by the historical education and training provision that the workforce are used to, the workforce's willingness to take it up, their preferences for particular modes of delivery, the opinions of others (e.g. the public and patients), current fashions (topics and type of delivery), and pressure from local champions or special interest groups.
4 Provision can be mapped out once plans have been agreed. Consider how to meet the needs of the entire workforce for generic knowledge and skills – for example, skills needed for interacting effectively with patients and the public, uni-professional education and training in specialty areas, inter-professional provision whenever appropriate and practicable, and managerial or organisational education and training for those whose roles and responsibilities indicate this.
5 Appraisal and evaluation of the skills, knowledge, attitudes and competence of the workforce with regard to the relevance to service needs should be a regular feature of any education and training programme, with feedback on achievements and gaps in provision at all stages in the cycle. The healthcare system will continue to develop and extend its focus of interest and capability, and any education and training programme should be proactive in this dynamic process, and capable of responding reactively to new directives and developments or public opinion.

EDUCATIONAL PLAN FOR A PRACTICE OR DIRECTORATE

Practice- or unit-based PDPs encompass the needs of the individual, the practice, the local healthcare organisation and the healthcare system in general.[3] Such a plan should include the needs of all healthcare providers and attached staff.

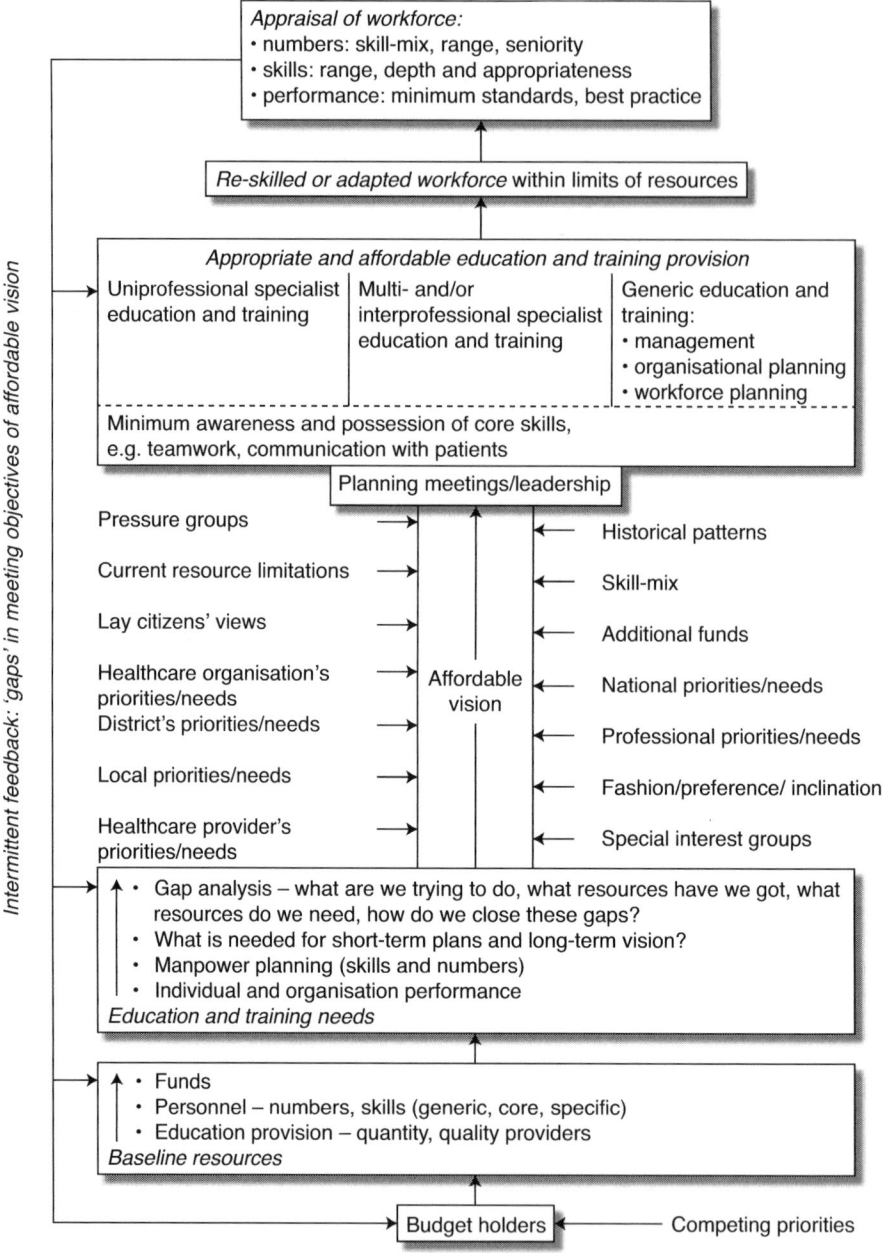

Appraisal of workforce:
• numbers: skill-mix, range, seniority
• skills: range, depth and appropriateness
• performance: minimum standards, best practice

Re-skilled or adapted workforce within limits of resources

Appropriate and affordable education and training provision

| Uniprofessional specialist education and training | Multi- and/or interprofessional specialist education and training | Generic education and training:
• management
• organisational planning
• workforce planning |

Minimum awareness and possession of core skills, e.g. teamwork, communication with patients

Planning meetings/leadership

Pressure groups → | ← Historical patterns

Current resource limitations → | ← Skill-mix

Lay citizens' views → | ← Additional funds

Healthcare organisation's priorities/needs → | Affordable vision | ← National priorities/needs

District's priorities/needs → | ← Professional priorities/needs

Local priorities/needs → | ← Fashion/preference/ inclination

Healthcare provider's priorities/needs → | ← Special interest groups

• Gap analysis – what are we trying to do, what resources have we got, what resources do we need, how do we close these gaps?
• What is needed for short-term plans and long-term vision?
• Manpower planning (skills and numbers)
• Individual and organisation performance
Education and training needs

• Funds
• Personnel – numbers, skills (generic, core, specific)
• Education provision – quantity, quality providers
Baseline resources

Budget holders ← Competing priorities

Intermittent feedback: 'gaps' in meeting objectives of affordable vision

FIGURE 3.1

EDUCATIONAL PLAN FOR INDIVIDUAL PRACTITIONERS

Assessment of your own or others' educational and training needs must include consideration of the differing priority areas of national bodies (e.g. the government), district bodies, your local organisation, your practice or unit and the general public. Decide how to weigh one priority against another, as education and training time is limited by competing service demands. Actively look at every educational or training event for an opportunity to make the activity as relevant as possible to healthcare needs as a whole. One way of doing this is to visualise the planned educational activity as shown in Figure 3.2a. If you 'join the dots' midway along those sides of the octagon that apply to any particular topic, the resulting surface area will give you a visual representation of the number of priority areas that the topic addresses.

In the octagon in Figure 3.2b, all of the dots are joined when the educational topic is 'coronary heart disease (CHD)', because this subject is part of any national strategy for prevention and management of CHD, and may also be a priority area of the district population (if standard mortality rates are relatively high), the practice, work colleagues and individual patients (if there has been a sudden death, or if there is particular interest in the quality of cardiac care as a work-based team), professional (if the focus is on the capability to resuscitate any person who arrests) and personal (if there is a wish to

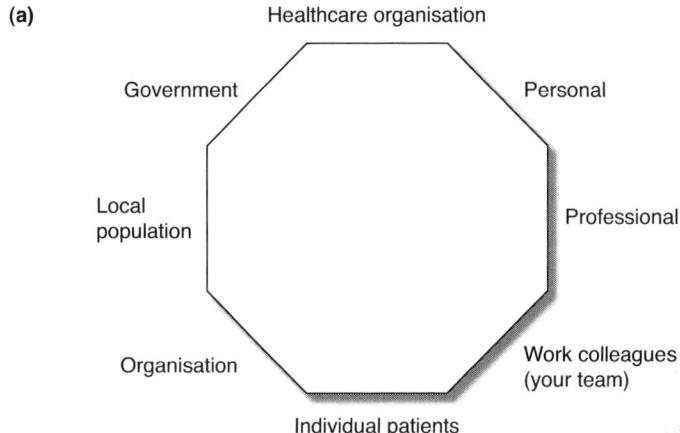

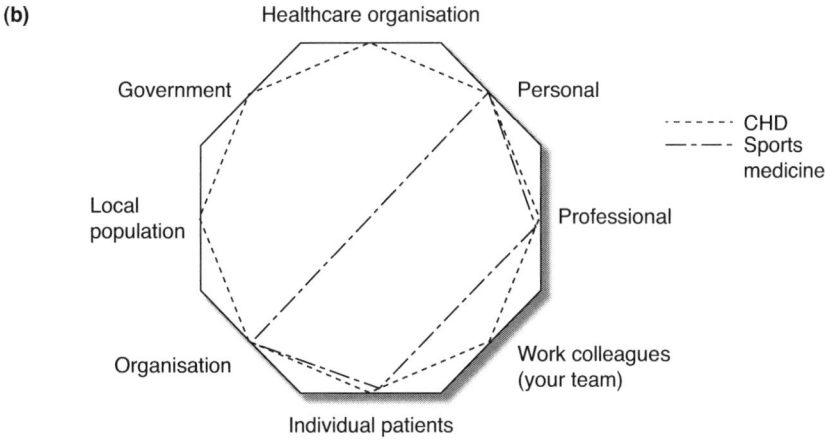

FIGURE 3.2

maintain competence in managing CHD and adopt best practice). The surface area that you obtain as a result of joining the dots gives you some idea of the number of priority areas that a potential educational topic addresses, but no idea of the need or baseline depth of knowledge. If the surface area that you draw out is relatively small, as in the second example ('sports medicine'), think how you might teach or learn about the topic so that it is more relevant to priority areas for development of others as well as yourself.

REFERENCES

1 Kennedy I. *The Bristol Royal Infirmary Inquiry. Final report.* London: Department of Health; 2001.
2 National Health Service Executive. *The New NHS: modern, dependable.* London: HMSO; 1997.
3 Calman K. *A Review of Continuing Professional Development in General Practice.* London: Department of Health; 1998.
4 Houghton G, Wall D. Clinical governance and the Chief Medical Officer's review of GP education: piecing the New NHS jigsaw together. *Med Teacher.* 1999; **21**: 5–6.
5 National Health Service Executive. *Working Together: securing a quality workforce for the NHS.* London: Department of Health; 1998.
6 Macleod N, Moloney R, Chambers R. *The Education and Training Needs of Primary Care Groups.* Stafford: Staffordshire University; 1999.
7 Greiner AC, Knebel E, Committee on the Health Professions Education Summit. *Health Professions Education: a bridge to quality.* Washington, DC: National Academies Press; 2003. www.acme-assn.org/valuable_resources/IOM-ABridgetoQuality.pdf
8 www.caipe.org.uk/about-us/defining-ipe/
9 Hammick M, Freeth D, Koppel I *et al.* A best evidence systematic review of interprofessional education. *Med Teacher.* 2007; **29**: 735–51.
10 Accreditation of Interprofessional Health Education. *Principles and Practices for Integrating Interprofessional Education into the Accreditation Standards for Six Health Professions in Canada.* www.afmc.ca/aiphe-afiss/documents/AIPHE_Principles_and_Implementation_Guide_EN.pdf
11 Standing Committee on Postgraduate Medical and Dental Education. *Multi-Professional Working and Learning: sharing the educational challenge.* London: SCOPME; 1997.
12 Standing Committee on Postgraduate Medical and Dental Education. *Continuing Professional Development for Doctors and Dentists.* London: SCOPME; 1998.
13 Health Canada. *Interprofessional Education for Collaborative Patient-Centred Practice.* www.hc-sc.gc.ca/hcs-sss/hhr-rhs/strateg/interprof/index-eng.php
14 Royal College of Nursing. *The Impact and Effectiveness of Inter-Professional Education in Primary Care: an RCN literature review.* London: Royal College of Nursing; 2006. www.rcn.org.uk/__data/assets/pdf_file/0004/78718/003091.pdf
15 Association of Faculties of Medicine of Canada. *Accreditation of Interprofessional Health Education.* Ottawa, ON: Association of Faculties of Medicine of Canada. www.afmc.ca/pdf/Accreditation%20of%20Interprofessional%20Health%20Education-e.pdf
16 Chambers R, Lucking A. Partners in time? Can PCGs really succeed where others have failed? *Br J Health Care Management.* 1998; **4**: 489–91.
17 Belbin RM. *Management Teams: why they succeed or fail.* Oxford: Heinemann; 1981.
18 World Federation for Medical Education. *Continuing Professional Development (CPD)*

of Medical Doctors: WFME global standards. Copenhagen: World Federation for Medical Education; 2003. www3.sund.ku.dk/Activities/WFME%20Standard%20Documents%20 and%20translations/WFME%20CPD.pdf

19 Roland M, Holden J, Campbell S. *Quality Assessment for General Practice: supporting clinical governance in primary care groups.* Manchester: National Primary Care Research and Development Centre, University of Manchester; 1999.

20 Academy of Medical Royal Colleges. *A Review of the Ten Principles for CPD in the Context of the Proposals of the Donaldson Report.* London: Academy of Medical Royal Colleges; 2007.

21 Nursing and Midwifery Council. *Standards for the Preparation and Practice of Supervisors of Midwives.* London: Nursing and Midwifery Council; 2006. www.nmc-uk.org/aDisplay Document.aspx?documentID=2229

22 Woodrow M. The struggle for the soul of lifelong learning. *Widening Particip Lifelong Learn.* 1999; **1**: 9–12.

23 Davies D. The learning society: moving on to the workplace. *Widening Particip Lifelong Learn.* 1999; **1**: 13–19.

24 Chambers R, Field S, Muller E. Educating GP non-principals. *Educ Gen Pract.* 1998; **9**: 108–64.

25 National Health Service Executive. *The New NHS: modern and dependable. Developing the education and workforce framework.* Working Paper. London: NHS Executive; 1999.

26 Chief Nursing Officer. *Integrating Theory and Practice in Nursing.* London: NHS Executive; 1998.

27 Regen E, Smith J, Shapiro J. *First Off the Starting Block: lessons from GP commissioning pilots for primary care groups.* Birmingham: Health Service Management Centre, University of Birmingham; 1999.

28 Wilson T, Butler F, Watson M. Establishing educational needs in a new organisation. *Career Focus, BMJ.* 1998; **317**: 2–3.

29 Syder B, Kent A. *Phoenix Agenda.* Leeds: NHS Executive; 1998.

30 Garcarz W. *Primary Care Group Formation: organisational development tools.* Birmingham: Birmingham Health Authority; 1998.

31 Garcarz W, Chambers R, Ellis S. *Make Your Healthcare Organisation a Learning Organisation.* Oxford: Radcliffe Medical Press; 2003.

32 Department of Health. *Workforce Development Confederations: functions, accountabilities and working relationships.* London: Department of Health; 2002.

FURTHER READING

- Accreditation of Interprofessional Health Education. *Principles and Practices for Integrating Interprofessional Education into the Accreditation Standards for Six Health Professions in Canada.* www.afmc.ca/aiphe-afiss/documents/AIPHE_Principles_and_Implementation_Guide_ EN.pdf
- Canadian Interprofessional Health Collaborative. www.cihc.ca
- Centre for the Advancement of Interprofessional Education. www.caipe.org.uk
- Chambers R, Wakley G, Iqbal Z et al. Multidisciplinary learning. In: *Prescription for Learning: techniques, games and activities.* Oxford: Radcliffe Medical Press; 2002.

CHAPTER 4

Educational concepts: the theory behind the practical aspects of teaching and learning

This chapter considers the following simplified concepts in education that will help you to understand how learners might learn and how you may function better as a teacher:
- ➤ psychology of learning
- ➤ educational climate
- ➤ constructivism
- ➤ experiential learning cycle
- ➤ learning styles
- ➤ educational cycle
- ➤ motivation.

THE PSYCHOLOGY OF LEARNING

In the first half of the twentieth century there were two main schools of thought about learning theory, namely behaviourist and cognitive. A third group, the motivational theorists, had less pre-eminence.[1]

The behaviourist school reflected a mechanistic view of teaching and learning – a given stimulus produces a certain reaction in the learner. A simple example is the rat in a box with a lever that, when pressed, releases food. The rat quickly learns the result of pressing the lever, and the action is thus reinforced. At a higher level, on a resuscitation course there may be a particular procedure to be learned, which if performed according to the manual is correct and if performed another way is incorrect. Candidates are taught to react in a certain way to specific situations, and not necessarily to think out their actions first. In emergency situations, where split-second reactions are important, this may be reasonable. Cognitive theorists rejected this mechanistic view and argued that individual learners were not passive organisms who responded to stimuli in a certain way, but rather that they thought about things, selected out and processed information, and then acted in different ways to altered circumstances. They believed that prior knowledge and skills were important and new ideas were built on old ones. Thus learners could reorganise their existing knowledge to solve new problems, and 'latent learning' – learning that takes place along the way and does not show itself until much later, when it is needed – could also occur.

Motivation of learners should also be considered. McGregor's 'Theory X and Theory Y' teaching strategies[2] (*see* Box 4.1) show how this influences the way in which we respond as teachers.

BOX 4.1 Theory X and Theory Y of learning[2]

- Theory X: learners are irresponsible and immature.
- Theory Y: learners are motivated and responsible.

Characteristics of Theory X
- Learners hate work and avoid it if they can.
- They need to be coerced to work by control, direction and punishment, or they need to be coerced by reward, praise and privileges.
- Learners wish to be directed, avoid any responsibility, have no ambition but want security.
- Few learners have any imagination, ingenuity or creativity.
- The intellect of the average learner is already all used up.

Characteristics of Theory Y
- Learning is a natural activity, and learners will try to succeed in achieving objectives to which they are committed.
- Commitment to learning is a function of rewards associated with that achievement.
- Learners learn to accept and seek out responsibility for their own learning.
- Most learners have imagination, ingenuity and creativity.
- The intellectual potential of the average learner is only partly utilised. There is a lot more in there!

The three main theories of learning – behavioural, cognitive and motivational – have been summarised and matched against 13 educational strategies (*see* Box 4.2).[1]

BOX 4.2 The three main theories of learning

Behaviourist mode
1 *Activity:* learning by doing, where active is better than passive learning (students will learn more when they are actively involved).
2 *Repetition, generalisation and discrimination:* frequent practice in a variety of situations helps (especially when learning new skills).
3 *Reinforcement:* positive is better than negative. Rewards, praise and successes are more effective reinforcers than failures.

Cognitive mode
4 *Learning with understanding:* meaningful and fits in with what learners already know.
5 *Organisation and structure:* logical and well-organised material is easier to follow and learn from.

6 *Perceptual features:* the way in which a problem is displayed to learners is important (e.g. a handout accompanying a lecture).

7 *Cognitive feedback:* it is important to know how well you are doing.

8 *Individual differences:* differences in ability, personality and motivation all affect learning.

Motivational mode

9 *Natural learning:* learners are naturally curious and learn from all kinds of situations.

10 *Purposes and goals:* learners have needs, goals and purposes, which are relevant to motivation in learning.

11 *Social situation:* the group atmosphere and whether there is cooperation or competition with others affects success and satisfaction in learning.

12 *Choice, relevance and responsibility:* learning is more effective when the material is relevant, chosen by the learners and delivered when they want to learn it.

13 *Anxiety and emotions:* when learning involves emotions, learning is more significant; it is most effective in a non-threatening environment.

EDUCATIONAL CLIMATE

Educationalists refer to the 'atmosphere' or 'ambience' of an organisation as the 'climate' or sometimes the 'press'. Knowles states that the first requirement for adult learning is to establish the physical and psychological climate or ethos with regard to learning.[3] Teachers must consider all aspects of the 'educational environment':

> The crucial knowledge concerns the overall atmosphere or characteristics of the classroom; the kind of things that are rewarded, encouraged, emphasised; the style of life that is valued in the classroom or school community and is most visibly expressed and felt.[4]

The educational climate may be subdivided into three parts:

1 physical environment (facilities, comfort, safety, food, shelter, etc.)

2 emotional climate (security, positive methods, reinforcement, etc.)

3 intellectual climate (learning with patients, reflective practice, evidence-based, up-to-date knowledge and skills).

Remember learners' likes and dislikes with regard to educational climate. Their likes include:

➤ encouragement and praise

➤ learning on the job

➤ discussing cases, including best management practice, a chance to present the case and describe their management

➤ challenge

➤ a relaxed atmosphere

➤ group discussions

➤ positive feedback

➤ approachable seniors who are up to date, enthusiastic about their subject and able to say 'I don't know, let's look it up.'

Dislikes include:
➤ just looking at mistakes
➤ humiliation, especially in front of patients and staff
➤ being shouted at
➤ being frightened
➤ teachers not appreciating that they have knowledge gaps
➤ irrelevant teaching about rare conditions
➤ senior colleagues who are out of date and unable to admit that they do not know everything.

The educational environment must be considered in healthcare, as it encourages important abstract behaviours such as 'professionalism' or 'bedside manner.' By giving attention to aspects of the learning environment and offering yourself as a role model, you can contribute to the likelihood that such behaviours will be fostered.

Consider the questions posed in Box 4.3 in relation to the environment that you cultivate for your learners.[4]

BOX 4.3 CUES (College and University Environment Scales) to the educational environment[4]

- Scholarship: what am I doing to encourage scholarly, intellectual and academic pursuits?
- Practicality: how much attention do I give to the pragmatic and the practical, and to business-like efficiency?
- Community: is there concern for fostering friendliness and a sense of community both between teacher and students and among students?
- Awareness: what do I do that might encourage the development of a sense of personal identity, self-expression and social responsibility?
- Propriety: to what extent do I place emphasis on the environment being a polite and considerate sort of place, where 'proper' behaviours are called for, and where there is some emphasis on rules and regulations?

CONSTRUCTIVISM

Constructivism describes learning as based on prior knowledge, and the teacher not as a transmitter of knowledge but rather as a guide who facilitates this integration. Learners 'construct' their own knowledge on the basis of what they already know. Teachers should provide learning opportunities that challenge previously held opinions and current understanding. Following the constructivist model involves engaging students actively in learning activities, probably in small group settings, performing tasks that are taken from life experiences. Adequate time must be given for reflection on new experiences. The acquisition of new knowledge follows in-depth examination, and involves active judgements by learners about when and how to modify their existing knowledge.

This process of reflection is prompted by new information, surprises or unexpected events, and can be of two kinds:[5]
1 *reflection in action*: this occurs immediately, as the 'ability to learn and develop continually by creatively applying current and past experience and reasoning to unfamiliar events whilst they are occurring.'[6]

2 *reflection on action*: this occurs later, as the 'process of thinking back on what happened in a past situation, what may have contributed to it, whether the actions taken were appropriate. and how this situation may affect future practice.'[6]

Reflection does not come naturally to all learners. Effective teachers encourage learners to look critically at both the learning process and outcomes to increase their level of self-directedness (*see* Chapter 5).

THE EXPERIENTIAL LEARNING CYCLE

Learning from experience can be powerful. The experiential learning cycle demonstrates the stages that learners must pass through for learning to be effective:
  1 action (having the experience)
  2 reflection (thinking about how it went)
  3 conclusion (integrating one's reflections with existing knowledge and information from other sources, and forming a conclusion about how it went)
  4 planning (deciding whether to do it the same or differently next time).

Learners tend to be more comfortable in one or other of the stages of the experiential learning cycle. Some like to be busy and have lots of new experiences, and will need teachers to encourage them to plan or reflect more. Others may tend to prevaricate and over-plan new activities, and may require a gentle push to start new projects. Yet others quickly draw conclusions from events, and may need encouragement to reflect fully on outcomes and integrate this with other opinions before reaching a conclusion. Finally, some learners think long and hard about past experiences and are paralysed by indecision about what to do next time. They need to be encouraged to reach and test a conclusion.

LEARNING STYLES

Different individuals learn in different ways and can alter the way in which they learn, depending on circumstances and subject matter.[1] Learners have preferences for certain kinds of information and ways of using that information to learn. Several models have been described, none of which is the 'correct' one. All of the models are useful when thinking about the concept of learning styles.

Honey and Mumford's four learning styles

Honey and Mumford have done an enormous amount of work on the type of activities through which different people learn best.[7] To determine your learning style you must complete a 10-minute, 80-item, self-assessment questionnaire. The outcome divides learners into four different styles, described below, which map directly on to the stages of the experiential learning cycle. Individuals may have a combination of two styles, possess features of all four styles in similar proportions, or may have the features of one style only.
➤ **Activists** like to be fully involved in new experiences, are open-minded, and are happy to try anything once, thriving on the challenge of new experiences, but soon get bored and want to move on to the next challenge. They are gregarious

and like to be the centre of attention. Activists learn best with new experiences, short activities, situations where they can be centre stage (e.g. chairing meetings, leading discussions), when they are allowed to generate new ideas, have a go at things or brainstorm ideas.

➤ **Reflectors** like to stand back, think about things thoroughly and collect a lot of information before reaching a conclusion. They are cautious, take a back seat in meetings and discussions, adopt a low profile, and appear tolerant and unruffled. When they do act it is by using the wide picture of their own and others' views. Reflectors learn best from situations where they are allowed to watch and think about activities, think before acting, carry out research first, review evidence, produce carefully constructed reports and reach decisions in their own time.

➤ **Theorists** like to adapt and integrate observations into logical maps and models, using step-by-step processes. They tend to be perfectionists, detached, analytical and objective, and reject anything that is subjective and flippant in nature or that involves lateral thinking. Theorists learn best from activities where there are plans, maps and models to describe what is going on, time to explore the methodology, structured situations with a clear purpose, and when they are offered complex situations to understand and are intellectually stretched.

➤ **Pragmatists** like to try out ideas, theories and techniques to see whether they work in practice. They will act quickly and confidently on ideas that attract them, and are impatient with ruminating and open-ended discussions. They are down-to-earth people who like problem solving and making practical decisions. Pragmatists learn best when there is an obvious link between the subject and their job. They enjoy trying out techniques with coaching and feedback, practical issues and real problems to solve, and when given the immediate chance to implement what has been learned.

It is useful to determine your own style so that if you have a trainee who has a very different style to yours, you can accommodate your differences. You may have a reflector–theorist learning pattern. If you have a new learner who is an activist, they may not respond to your ideas, principles, maps and models of things. They may get bored easily and will want to proceed with the task and try new experiences. Unless you realise what is going on, you may not realise why conflict may arise.

Convergent and divergent thinkers

➤ **Convergent thinkers** tend to find a single solution to a problem that is presented to them.

➤ **Divergent thinkers** tend to generate new ideas, expand ideas and explore widely.

IQ tests do not measure all aspects of intelligence. They only test convergent thinking, and divergent thinking is not tested at all. There is a possible link between convergent thinking and science students, and divergent thinking and arts students. Teachers may react better to convergent thinkers, perceiving divergent thinkers as being more difficult to deal with. This does not seem to be a fixed learning style, and some change is possible, perhaps by the use of brainstorming sessions.

Serialists and holists

➤ **Serialists** learn best by taking one step at a time.
➤ **Holists** learn best by first obtaining the big picture and then filling in the steps.

Individuals appear to learn best when teaching is matched to their learning style. Some people are able to use either approach. Therefore if you expect learners to make their own way through learning material, it needs to be arranged so that it can be followed by both serialists and holists.

Deep and surface processors

➤ **Deep processors** like to focus on the main points of an article in order to understand it.
➤ **Surface processors** like to read through the material, remembering as much as possible.

Many students have great difficulty in summarising the main points in a text. Studies on the reading and summarising of text have suggested that deep processors look for the main ideas and principles and can summarise text well. Surface processors read through the text from start to finish and often fail to grasp the main points.

Deep and surface approaches to learning will be effective in different settings. Most learners know the difference and will adopt whichever approach seems appropriate. However, some learners will always adopt a surface approach because of their understanding of learning. The development of this understanding can be described in five stages.

1 Learning is understood by the learner to be an increase in knowledge – something done to the learner by the teacher.
2 Learning is memorising – the learner actively memorises information but does not transform it in any way.
3 Learning is the acquisition of facts and procedures to be used.
4 Learning is making sense – the learner makes an active search for abstract meaning.
5 Learning is understanding reality – knowledge acquired by the learner enables them to see the world differently.

Learners who understand learning at a surface level (levels 1–3) are unlikely to take a deep approach to learning. Unsurprisingly, a relationship exists between understanding of learning and expectations of teaching. Learners in the reproducing group (levels 1–3) expect teaching to be 'closed' (i.e. teachers select the content, present it to the learners and then test them to see whether it has 'stuck'). Learners in the 'making sense' levels (levels 4–5) feel that teaching should be 'open' (i.e. the learner functions independently, with facilitation).

Often learners are at levels 1–3 simply because they have only been exposed to closed teaching, especially that involved in exam preparation. Assessment systems can dictate the way in which learners learn. Development of tasks that make different demands on learners can develop their understanding of what learning is.

The characteristics of learning activities that could foster a surface approach to learning include:
➤ heavy workload

➤ relatively high number of teacher contact hours
➤ excessive amounts of course material
➤ lack of time to pursue subjects in depth
➤ lack of choice with regard to subject matter and study methods
➤ a threatening and anxiety-provoking assessment system.

How you can help learners to find approaches that suit their own styles

There are four main approaches to tailoring learning to individual needs:
➤ **Matching:** introverts (who are internally referenced) do better with well-structured situations, whereas extroverts (whose locus of stimulation is external to themselves) do better with less structured situations.
➤ **Allowing choice:** since learners come from a range of backgrounds and have different ways of learning and varying aims, you should aim for flexibility in your provision.
➤ **Providing several different methods of learning on the same course:** that way learners can mix and match, or will always find something that suits them.
➤ **Independent study:** complete freedom to study, whilst threatening to those that need structure, can give good results, especially with more mature learners.

THE EDUCATIONAL CYCLE

The principles of the educational cycle are applicable to many teaching and learning situations within healthcare education. The cycle can be used in a simple form, namely the 'training triangle' of *aims, methods* and *assessment*.[8] This educational cycle is a four-step model:

1 assessment of the individual's needs
2 setting educational objectives
3 choosing and using a variety of methods of teaching and learning
4 assessing whether learning has occurred.

Assessment of the individual's needs

What does the learner need to know? Assess what the learner has done before and knows about already while making reference to the appropriate training curriculum. Encourage the learner to use a tool to self-rate their levels of knowledge and skills in various areas. Using this, you may agree with your learner some key topics that they need to address during their time with you. You are now ready to progress to the next step of the cycle.

Setting educational objectives

Educational objectives are things that the learner will be able to do at the end of the course, often written in behavioural terms. For many educational activities, the objectives model fits very well, particularly in terms of practical skills. Once the learner and teacher have consulted the curriculum and have assessed needs, they can devise and agree a plan, listing a set of learning objectives to be achieved.

Remember that assessment begins with the setting of learning objectives.

Choosing and using a variety of methods of teaching and learning

There is no single teaching method that is best. Different methods suit different situations, learners and teachers. However, there are optimum methods for teaching different things (*see* Chapter 8).

Most people learn best by 'doing', using active methods of learning, rather than sitting passively in a lecture theatre. This is not news – it was recognised by an ancient Chinese proverb:

> I hear and I forget
>
> I see and I remember
>
> I do and I understand.

Assessing whether learning has occurred

How do you know whether learning has occurred? One simple approach is to base assessments (*see* Chapter 14) on learning objectives set at the beginning. If you have established good, achievable learning objectives and chosen appropriate learning methods, the learner will progress through the course and learn what you expected. So after setting learning objectives at the start, check the learner's progress using regular appraisal meetings, and assess completion of learning at the end.

MOTIVATION

Motivation is 'that within the individual, rather than without, which incites him or her to action.'[9] Motivation may be positive or negative.

Positive motivation makes you keen to learn about a subject because of an inspiring teacher, because the subject interests you, or because you can see its relevance to your future career.

Negative motivation makes you do things because of fear of failure, punishment or other adverse outcomes if you do not do something.

Positive motivation tends to lead to deeper understanding and better long-term learning than negative methods, which can lead to superficial learning that is often forgotten.

Motivation seems to be a basic human function. We seek to achieve things, to accept challenges, and to work at learning new ideas and new skills throughout our lives. In this area we may assume four principles of motivation:

1 We all have an inbuilt urge to attempt to achieve things.
2 Our needs are related to specific goals. Factors such as self-image, group bonding and security are all relevant.
3 The relationship between needs and goals is complex and unstable. The same needs produce different behaviours in different individuals.
4 We all have many needs, but only a few are subject to conscious action at any one time.

Intrinsic and extrinsic factors influence motivation. Intrinsic factors come from within the individual, and include wanting to succeed at something, achieving a career goal, satisfying curiosity and accepting a challenge. Such intrinsic motivational forces may be very strong. Extrinsic factors, from outside influences, include competition, respect for others, not wishing to let the side down, and admiration of one's peers. Extrinsic motivational forces may be positive or negative. Competition among students may be helpful to some but may demotivate others, especially with regard to many types of assessment. These may produce an underlying fear and anxiety, which force the student to learn a certain amount in order to pass the test, but the material is often learned superficially and soon forgotten.

Motivational theory: Maslow's hierarchy of needs[10]

Maslow's motivational theory[10] described a hierarchy of needs, with the most basic needs at the bottom and the more social and self-realisation needs higher up. Physiological needs, such as food, clothing and shelter, are necessary for any living creature to survive. Safety and security issues come next, and are related to the survival needs lower down in the hierarchy. However, for most people these needs are usually well satisfied, and therefore rarely help to motivate them.

Despite these issues, higher needs, the self-realisation needs ('doing your own thing'), are much more powerful motivating factors in today's world. In between these needs at the top and the bottom of the pyramid are two needs that are controversially placed in Maslow's hierarchy (*see* Figure 4.1).

First, social needs are positioned lower than esteem needs, but for many people esteem needs are considerably higher than social ones. Social needs are related to being part of a group, belonging, being loved, and so on. Esteem, on the other hand, refers to the need to be recognised, to be valued for one's own uniqueness, abilities and achievements. Thus there may be difficulties in reconciling these two needs. To quote Mr Spock, 'Are the needs of the many different from the needs of the one?'[11]

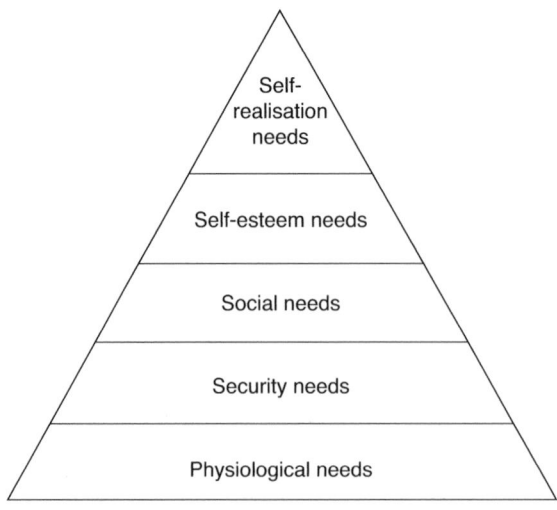

FIGURE 4.1

Tips from experienced teachers

Here are some practical ideas, drawn from the theories described in this chapter, about how you can motivate your trainees to learn more, be enthusiastic learners, and take control of and responsibility for their own learning.

- Think of positive ways to motivate your learners. What matters to them?
- Make learning interesting.
- Make learners active contributors to the learning process.
- Make learning relevant to learners' needs.
- Give regular constructive feedback on progress.
- Allow time, and build the skills required, for reflection.
- Reinforce positive aspects, not negative ones.
- Learning feeds on success.
- Give students responsibility for learning.
- Ensure that the right learning environment is provided.
- Reward good performance and good discipline.
- Goals should be translated into specific objectives.

And a final reminder – good teaching equals good motivation!

Other problems with the Maslow hierarchy include determining where money fits in. The lower needs, such as physiological, safety and security issues, are physical needs and therefore require money to satisfy them. In contrast, the next levels, such as esteem and social needs, seem to be psychological, with self-realisation at the top, which may not require expenditure of money. In a modified version of Maslow's hierarchy (*see* Figure 4.2), esteem and social needs have been combined on the same level, as it is difficult to distinguish which is higher than the other in this order. Self-realisation, which

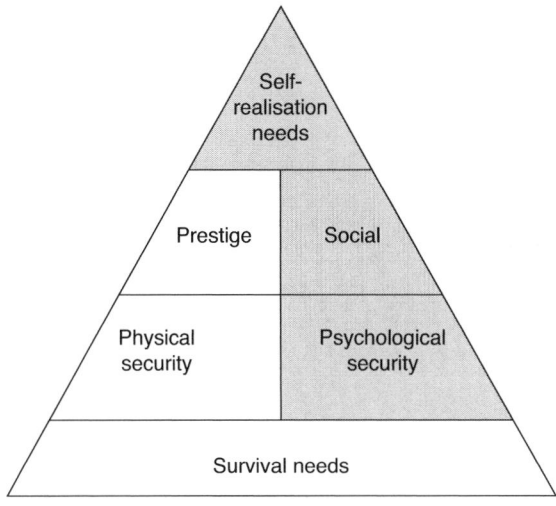

FIGURE 4.2

is still the primary motivation and continues to be purely psychological, remains at the top. The clear areas on the diagram are those that require monetary expenditure if they are to be achieved. The shaded areas are the psychological ones, such as trust in your teachers, confidence in your organisation, the educational climate in your institution, and so on.

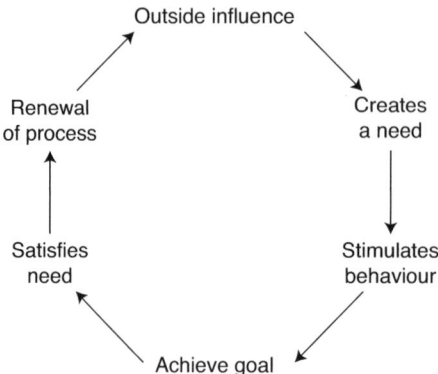

FIGURE 4.3

The motivational cycle

The motivational cycle (*see* Figure 4.3) may be of help in understanding where learners are in a particular situation.

REFERENCES

1 Beard RM, Hartley J. *Teaching and Learning in Higher Education*. 4th edn. Newcastle upon Tyne: Athaeneum Press; 1984.
2 McGregor D. *The Human Side of Experience*. New York: McGraw-Hill; 1960.
3 Knowles MS. *Androgogy in Action: applying modern principles of adult learning*. San Francisco, CA: Jossey-Bass; 1984.
4 Pace CR. *College and University Environmental Scales. Technical manual*. Princeton, NJ: Education Testing Service; 1963.
5 Schon DA. *Educating the Reflective Practitioner: toward a new design for teaching and learning in the professions*. San Francisco, CA: Jossey-Bass; 1987.
6 Kauffman DM. Applying educational theory in practice. ABC of learning and teaching. *BMJ.* 2003; **326:** 213–16.
7 Honey P, Mumford A. *Using Your Learning Styles*. Maidenhead: Peter Honey; 1986.
8 Pereira Gray DJ. *Training for General Practice*. Plymouth: MacDonald and Evans; 1982.
9 Peyton JWR. *Teaching and Learning in Medical Practice*. Rickmansworth: Manticore Europe; 1998.
10 Maslow AH. *Motivation and Personality*. New York: Harper and Row; 1970.
11 Mr Spock. *Star Trek II*. Paramount Pictures; 1982.

FURTHER READING

- Foundation for Advancement of International Medical Education and Research (FAIMER). Educational tools available at www.faimer.org/links/educators.html#edtools
- Learning-Theories.com contains an index of learning theories and models at www.learning -theories.com
- Scaling the Heights. Educational resources available at www.resources.scalingtheheights. com
- The Theory Into Practice (TIP) database contains over 50 one-page summaries of important educational concepts at http://tip.psychology.org

CHAPTER 5

Adult learning and
self-directed learners

Healthcare professionals are expected to be 'adult learners' – they will be independent and self-directed. Knowles coined the term 'androgogy' to refer to the art and science of teaching adults.[1]

Adult learning theory is built on five assumptions.[1]

1 Adults are independent and self-directing.
2 They have accumulated a great deal of experience, which is a rich resource for learning.
3 They value learning that integrates with the demands of their everyday life.
4 They are more interested in immediate, problem-centred approaches than in subject-centred ones.
5 They are more motivated to learn by internal drivers than by external ones.

Healthcare is too broad for all the content to be delivered by teachers. You must equip your learners with the skills to solve problems and continue learning throughout their careers:

> Education teaches us to solve problems, the nature of which may not be known to us at the time the education is taking place, and the solutions to which cannot be seen or even imagined by our teachers.[2]

Many people are frustrated by learners who do not behave as adults and expect to be 'spoon-fed.' Underlying this frustration is often a failure to recognise that the capacity to be self-directed is not an all-or-nothing function that develops overnight. Learners act at different levels or stages of self-direction depending on, for example, previous teaching, learning and assessment experiences, the subject matter and context of learning. Not all learners are ready to take responsibility for their own learning.

Effective teachers recognise this and realise that adult learning is *facilitated* by the teacher. Consider learning to be like a voyage in a boat. As the teacher you do not stop being the rudder, but you avoid being the oars. Brookfield has debated the subject of adult learning at length, providing many examples.[3]

GROW'S STAGES OF SELF-DIRECTED LEARNING (SSDL) MODEL

Grow's SSDL model builds on work by Hersey, and is a helpful way to look at tensions that can arise if the learner's and teacher's levels are not matched.[4] With kind permission of the author to use his illustrations, the essential features of this model are reproduced below.

The SSDL model describes four developmental stages for students (S1–4):
1 dependent learner
2 interested learner
3 involved learner
4 self-directed learner

and four styles of teaching (T1–4):
1 authority, coach
2 motivator, guide
3 facilitator
4 consultant, delegator.

Grow has depicted these four types of teaching with the following four cartoons:

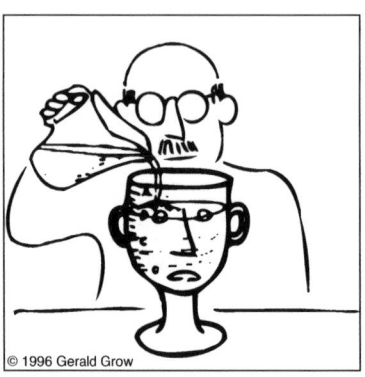

© 1996 Gerald Grow

T1 TEACHER

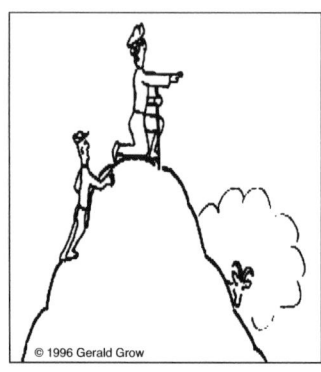

© 1996 Gerald Grow

T3 TEACHER

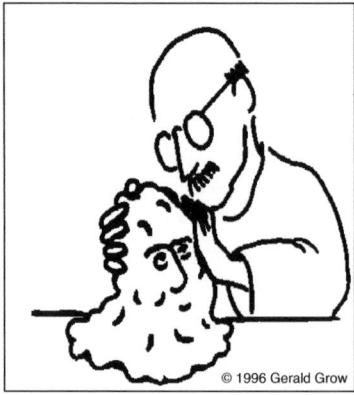

© 1996 Gerald Grow

T2 TEACHER

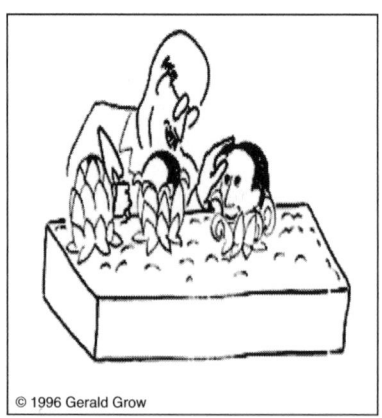

© 1996 Gerald Grow

T4 TEACHER

For each learning stage, some ways of delivering teaching and activities are better suited than others (*see* Table 5.1).

Tensions can arise if the learner's stage and delivery of teaching are mismatched – for example, when dependent learners are placed with non-directive teachers and when self-directed learners work with highly directive teachers (*see* Table 5.2).

T1/S4 mismatch

When self-directed students (S4) are paired with an authoritarian teacher (T1), problems may arise, although some S4 learners develop the ability to function well and retain overall control of their learning, even under directive teachers. However, other S4 learners will resent the authoritarian teacher and rebel against the barrage of low-level demands. This mismatch may cause the learner to rebel or to retreat into boredom.

Furthermore, the T1 teacher will probably not interpret such rebellion as the result of a mismatch. Instead that teacher is likely to see the learner as surly, uncooperative and unprepared to concentrate on learning basic facts. Extreme over-control by any leader results in stress and conflict, and in the follower engaging in behaviour designed to get the leader out – or to escape from under the leader.

T1/S3-S4 mismatch

Learners who are capable of more individual involvement in learning are relegated to passive roles in authoritarian classrooms.

Adults who return to education may find themselves in this position. Their life experiences and learning skills generally enable them to learn at the S3 or S4 level,

TABLE 5.1 Stages of development of learning and teaching, leading to self-directed learning

Stage or level of development of learner	Learner	Teacher	Examples of teaching activities
Stage 1	Dependent	Authority, coach	Coaching with immediate feedback Drill Informational lecture Overcoming deficiencies and resistance
Stage 2	Interested	Motivator, guide	Inspiring lecture plus guided discussion Goal-setting and learning strategies
Stage 3	Involved	Facilitator	Discussion facilitated by teacher who participates as equal Seminar Group projects
Stage 4	Self-directed	Consultant, delegator	Dissertation Individual work or self-directed study group

TABLE 5.2 Mismatch of levels of self-direction of learning with type of delivery of teaching

	T1: Authority Expert	T2: Motivator	T3: Facilitator	T4: Delegator
S4: Self-directed learner	Severe mismatch Students resent authoritarian teacher	*Mismatch*	Near match	Match
S3: Involved learner	*Mismatch*	Near match	Match	Near match
S2: Interested learner	Near match	Match	Near match	*Mismatch*
S1: Dependent learner	Match	Near match	*Mismatch*	Severe mismatch Learners resent freedom they are not ready for

but they may be placed with teachers accustomed to using Stage 1 and 2 methods on adolescents.

Furthermore, after many years of responsibility, adults may experience difficulty learning from T1 teachers. Adults may be accustomed to having authority, and unused to blindly doing what they are told without understanding why and consenting to the task.

Adults returning for postgraduate study, in particular, may run aground on courses like statistics, which are often taught by briskly directive teachers using the Stage 1 mode. The more appropriate Stage 3 mode is not always used with older learners when teachers lack experience in this type of teaching.

T4/S1 mismatch

When dependent learners (S1) are paired with a T3 or T4 teacher, they may be delegated responsibility for learning that they are not equipped to handle.

Such learners may be unable to make use of the 'freedom to learn' because they lack the following necessary skills for self-directed learning:
➤ goal setting
➤ self-evaluation
➤ project management
➤ critical thinking
➤ group participation
➤ learning strategies
➤ information resources
➤ self-esteem.

Learners may resent the teacher for forcing upon them a freedom for which they are not ready. These dependent learners expect close supervision, immediate feedback, frequent interaction, constant motivation, and the reassuring presence of an authority-figure telling them what to do. Such learners are unlikely to respond well to the delegating style of teaching, a hands-off delegator, or a critical theorist who demands that they confront their own learning roles.

Grow describes the results of this mismatch as a kind of 'havoc' that occurs when the followers do not receive the guidance that they need, and:

> lacking the ability to perform the task, [they] tend to feel that the leader has little interest in their work and does not care about them personally. [This form of teacher leadership makes] it difficult for these followers to increase their ability, and reinforces their lack of confidence. If the leader waits too long but then provides high amounts of structure, the followers tend to see this action as a punitive rather than a helping relationship.[4]

The learner's stage of self-direction is often a result of the teaching that they have previously experienced. Consider the following:

> I am the product of a system built around assignments, deadlines, and conventional examinations. Therefore, with this course graded by the flexible method and four other courses graded by the more conventional methods, I tend to give less attention to this course than it merits, due to a lack of well-defined requirements.

This learner has made a strategic decision about study. Other learners in this position may experience shock and resentment when faced with the necessity of making unguided, responsible choices.

The false Stage 4 learner

Some students appear to be Stage 4 self-directed learners, but turn out to be highly dependent students in a state of defiance. The one who shouts loudest, 'No! I'll do it *my* way!' is likely to be a 'false independent' learner who may resist mastering the necessary details of the subject and 'wing it' at an abstract level.

False independent learners need help to raise their knowledge and skills to the level of their self-belief. They may need to master how to learn productively from others, and may benefit from a strong-willed teacher who challenges them to become autonomous and effective.

Dependent, resistant learners as a product of the educational system

The way in which undergraduates are often taught can produce learners who resist direction. A group of highly resistant learners can coerce teachers into an authoritarian mode, and then frustrate them, at the same time being dependent on teachers and resentful of being taught.

The resistant form of Stage 1 is probably not a natural condition. It results from years of dependency training. Most children are naturally Stage 3 or 4 learners when undirected. Even when taught in a directive manner, they are generally available, interested and excitable, and have a spontaneous creative energy that they are willing to direct into satisfying projects under the guidance of a capable teacher.

Resistant dependent learning may be a product of culture and upbringing, as well as of the education system. Sources of resistance in adult learners may include threats to cultural identity that might have been generated by the (hopefully now changing) pressures of hierarchical medicine. You need to understand dependency in context – certain forms of help may make the problem worse.

Using the SSDL model in practice

As outlined above, the SSDL model describes four styles of teaching (T1-4). Teaching styles and application of the theory underlying teaching and learning styles are explored further in Chapter 6.

KNOWLES' GUIDELINES ON TEACHING SELF-DIRECTED ADULTS

Knowles defined seven fundamentals that have stood the test of time as guidelines to encourage adult learners:[1]

1 Establish an effective learning climate in which learners feel safe and comfortable expressing themselves.
2 Involve learners in mutual planning of relevant methods and curricular content.
3 Trigger internal motivation by involving learners in diagnosing their own needs.
4 Give learners more control by encouraging them to formulate their own learning objectives.
5 Encourage learners to identify resources and devise strategies for using resources to achieve their objectives.
6 Support learners in carrying out their learning plans.
7 Develop learners' skills of critical reflection by involving them in evaluating their own learning.

Following these guidelines might encourage learners to move up through the stages.

BROOKFIELD'S PRINCIPLES OF ADULT LEARNING

There are six principles of adult learning that you should build into your teaching.[3]

1 **Participation is voluntary** – the decision to learn is that of the learner.
2 **There should be mutual respect** – shown by teachers and learners for each other, and by learners for other learners.
3 **Collaboration is important** – between learners and teachers, and among learners.
4 **Action and reflection** – learning is a continuous process of investigation, exploration, action, reflection and further action.
5 **Critical reflection** – this brings awareness that alternatives can be presented as challenges to the learner to gather evidence, ask questions and develop a critically aware frame of mind.
6 **Self-directed adult individuals need to be nurtured.**

HOW TO PUT THE PRINCIPLES OF ADULT LEARNING INTO PRACTICE

What can busy healthcare professionals do to help themselves and their learners to develop into self-directed, independent adult learners? Brookfield gives ten tips on doing this (*see* Box 5.1).

BOX 5.1 How to create an adult learner

1 Progressively reduce the learner's dependence on the teachers.
2 Help the learner to understand the use of learning resources, including the experiences of fellow learners.
3 Help the learner to use reflective practice to define their learning needs.
4 Help the learner to define their learning objectives, plan their programmes and assess their own progress.
5 Organise what is to be learned in terms of personal understanding, goals and concerns at the learner's level of understanding.
6 Encourage the learner to take decisions, and to expand their learning experiences and range of opportunities for learning.
7 Encourage the use of criteria for judging all aspects of learning, not just those that are easy to measure.
8 Facilitate problem posing and problem solving in relation to personal and group needs issues.
9 Reinforce progressive mastery of skills through constructive feedback and mutual support.
10 Emphasise experiential learning (learning by doing, learning on the job) and use of learning contracts.

WORK-BASED LEARNING

Work-based learning aligns with the principles of adult learning, and represents the most accessible opportunities for self-directed learning during clinical work. Clinical experiences offer a vast range of learning opportunities. Encourage self-directed work-based learning by promoting and enhancing the quality of:

➤ reflection
➤ management of complaints
➤ significant events and critical incidents
➤ audit
➤ handover.

Reflection

All healthcare practitioners and teachers should regularly reflect on their practice. Processes of reflection, including *reflection in action* and *reflection on action*,[5] were introduced in Chapter 4. Formal evidence of reflection is required for clinical and academic professional portfolios, and these skills are often sought in job recruitment processes. Learners sometimes struggle to see the worth of reflection and, anecdotally, this can be a problem among undergraduates. You must undertake regular reflection on your own work, be able to assist learners with reflection, and highlight the benefits of doing so.

Why reflect?

The important benefits of reflection are as follows:

➤ keeping abreast of changes to the healthcare system, patient expectations and/or medical knowledge

➤ helping to understand why things went well or why they didn't – this can help both clinical practice and self-esteem, particularly if things have gone wrong

➤ helping you to make sense of a difficult situation, to prevent a knee-jerk reaction and unfair attribution of causation

➤ improving practice for the next time by taking a more informed and thought-out approach

➤ identifying learning needs to direct progress with personal development plans.

Although documented evidence of formal reflective practice is usually required, not all reflection needs to be written down. Take learners through the process of reflection through discussion (e.g. of a specific case or after role play).

Models of reflection

Reflection is about dissecting a situation and understanding the whys and the hows, rather than just stating what happened. A number of models outline stages of reflection:

➤ Gibbs' model of reflection (1988)[6]

➤ Johns' model of reflection (1994)[7]

➤ Atkins and Murphy's model of reflection (1994)[8]

➤ Holm and Stephenson's model of reflection (1994).[9]

Figure 5.1 summarises the key points from each to provide a cycle of prompts and processes that should be considered for effective reflection. However, not all of them may be applicable in every case.

Study as cases or questions arise

Reflection in action can be encouraged by teachers until it becomes self-directed. For example, in the clinical environment a learner may detect a condition that they have little experience of managing. Rather than stepping in and taking over, you can establish what the learner already knows and encourage them to address any knowledge gaps. Learners could trial a management approach or research missing knowledge in the clinical setting (e.g. by consulting evidence-based guidelines). This helps the learner to reach a conclusion through careful reasoning. The learner can direct their subsequent personal study to read up about their case and any remaining knowledge deficits. Maintaining a notebook to record questions, uncertainties or knowledge gaps may ensure that personal study can be directed appropriately.[10]

Following up cases that have been seen

To promote *reflection on action* and to prevent worthwhile reflective cases or situations being missed, learners should be encouraged to follow up cases that they have seen. Often the cases in which unforeseen circumstances arose are those from which the most can be learned. This may not necessarily mean that a mistake occurred, but rather that a patient's condition was not what it first appeared to be, or problems within healthcare system delivery prevented the originally planned management. Such cases may not be routinely brought to the attention of the learner if no mistakes were made or the patient has not been harmed. However, for the learner there may be a wealth of learning opportunities to address. The self-directed learner will take note of the patients they see and find out what subsequently happens during the care episode. Any cases

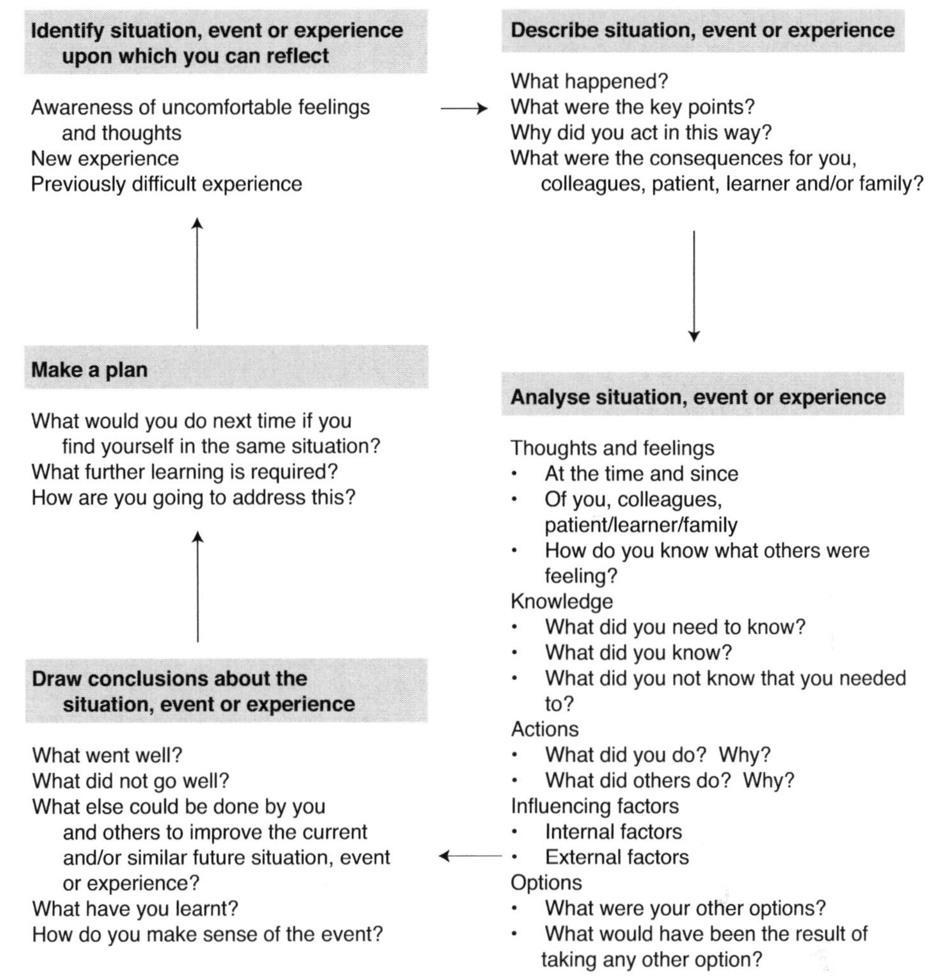

Identify situation, event or experience upon which you can reflect	Describe situation, event or experience

Identify situation, event or experience upon which you can reflect

Awareness of uncomfortable feelings and thoughts
New experience
Previously difficult experience

$\longrightarrow$

Describe situation, event or experience

What happened?
What were the key points?
Why did you act in this way?
What were the consequences for you, colleagues, patient, learner and/or family?

Make a plan

What would you do next time if you find yourself in the same situation?
What further learning is required?
How are you going to address this?

Analyse situation, event or experience

Thoughts and feelings
• At the time and since
• Of you, colleagues, patient/learner/family
• How do you know what others were feeling?
Knowledge
• What did you need to know?
• What did you know?
• What did you not know that you needed to?
Actions
• What did you do? Why?
• What did others do? Why?
Influencing factors
• Internal factors
• External factors
Options
• What were your other options?
• What would have been the result of taking any other option?

Draw conclusions about the situation, event or experience

What went well?
What did not go well?
What else could be done by you and others to improve the current and/or similar future situation, event or experience?
What have you learnt?
How do you make sense of the event?

$\longleftarrow$

FIGURE 5.1

in which unforeseen circumstances arose could be used for a significant event analysis (see below).

Complaints

You may feel defensive, disheartened and/or defeated upon receiving a complaint. However, complaints can be a useful stimulus for reflection and professional development. All professionals have to answer complaints that arise against them. As a junior, this may consist of providing a statement to senior staff, who may handle the situation from then on, or a formal response may be required. The skills learned through developing your reflective practice will assist with the production of such documents and also with the explanations that are provided to patients.

Maintaining a complaints record aids detection of any patterns of problems.[11] You should help learners to consolidate what they have learned from a complaint by considering the following:[12]

➤ description of the event
➤ concerns expressed by the complainant
➤ assessment of the complaint
➤ actions resulting from the assessment
➤ outcome, including the response to the complainant
➤ reflection on the experience and description of the learner's own involvement.

Significant events and critical incidents

Significant event analyses and critical incident reporting are increasingly becoming ingrained in the normal working practice of every healthcare professional, and are recognised conduits for identifying problems in services, initiating change to improve the quality of practice and patient safety, and influencing professional development through reflective learning.[12,13]

Significant events are cases in which an adverse, unforeseen or undesired (clinical, administrative or teaching) event has occurred. Often they involve situations in which harm or potential harm has resulted, but they do not necessarily do so. Therefore significant event analysis, which is a qualitative method of clinical audit that is undertaken on an individual case basis, has become a core component of work for many healthcare professionals, and is commonly required for appraisal, revalidation and professional accreditation.[14] Although the term 'critical incident' may be synonymous with 'significant event', it can also describe situations that the professional has identified as being important in their professional development. Thus the event may not have posed a threat to patient safety, but may have been challenging or particularly rich in learning points. The latter situation should be addressed in the same manner as reflection (*see* Figure 5.1).

The following steps are involved in significant event analysis:[14,15]
1 Identify the significant event for analysis.
2 Collect and collate data. This includes both factual information and gathering the thoughts, opinions and impressions of those involved.
3 Organise a meeting of relevant team members to discuss and analyse the significant event.
4 Agree and implement changes and organise follow-up.
5 Keep a written record.
6 Obtain peer review of the process and outcomes.

Formal reporting and analysis of significant events and critical incidents, like the management of complaints, are tasks that require good reflective skills, and are useful catalysts for learning. The same prompts can be used during steps 2–4 of a significant event analysis as are provided for reflection (*see* Figure 5.1). However, the involved team must participate in discussions and analysis of the event. Evidence that changes have occurred and the results of these changes are also usually required when reporting significant events, particularly for appraisal or revalidation purposes.[12]

Audit

Audit is the process whereby actual practice (organisational, clinical or educational) is compared with pre-defined standards and/or expectations of practice. In contrast to the individual case nature of significant event analysis, audits examine data of multiple cases, procedures or actions in order to obtain an overview of service provision. Data regarding your personal or service's practice are gathered and compared with the expected, pre-defined standards, and any deficits are identified. Formal reflection can help to explain areas that require attention and/or improvement to better meet the standards, and a plan should be made to initiate change. Once the change has been initiated, the whole process should be repeated to establish signs of improvement in adherence to expected practice. Thus a cycle is created that should be worked round repeatedly. You should assist your learners to undertake audit, and you should audit your own clinical and/or educational practice. Information on assessment of audits undertaken by others can be found in Chapter 14.

Handovers

Handovers are an excellent opportunity for work-based learning. They affect clinical care, and due to shortened working hours they have become increasingly frequent. Handovers can be the weak link of the patient care chain. Failure to hand over adequately can result in medical errors, wasted time and/or money, poor patient care, patient dissatisfaction and potentially patient death. Help learners to identify areas for development through robust and informative handover processes. Formal handovers involving seniors at each shift change provide an ideal platform for ensuring appropriate and adequate handover by junior staff, and for questioning and exploring patient management.

Tips from experienced teachers

Consistent reflection is the single most important skill to impart to a learner. It will lead to a change in attitudes as well as updated knowledge and new technical skills, and will enable them to maintain a consistently good performance throughout their health professional career.

REFERENCES

1 Knowles MS. *Androgogy in Action: applying modern principles of adult learning.* San Francisco, CA: Jossey-Bass; 1984.
2 Marinker M. Assessment of postgraduate medical education – future directions. In: Lawrence M and Pritchard P, eds. *General Practice Education: UK and Nordic perspectives.* London: Springer Verlag; 1992.
3 Brookfield SD. *Understanding and Facilitating Adult Learning.* Milton Keynes: Open University Press; 1986.
4 Grow GO. Teaching learners to be self-directed. *Adult Educ Quart.* 1996; **41**(3): 125–49.
5 Schon DA. *Educating the Reflective Practitioner: toward a new design for teaching and learning in the professions.* San Francisco, CA: Jossey-Bass; 1987.
6 Gibbs G. *Learning by Doing: a guide to teaching and learning methods.* Oxford: Further Education Unit, Oxford Polytechnic; 1988.
7 Johns C. Framing learning through reflection within Carper's fundamental ways of knowing in nursing. *J Adv Nurs.* 1995; **22**: 226–34.
8 Atkins S, Murphy K. Reflective practice. *Nurs Stand.* 1994; **8**: 49–56.
9 Palmer A, Burns S, Bulman C, eds. *Reflective Practice in Nursing: the growth of the professional practitioner.* Oxford: Blackwell Scientific Publications; 1994.

10 Johnson C, Bird J. *How to Teach Reflective Practice*. Cardiff: Cardiff University School of Postgraduate Medical and Dental Education. www.cardiff.ac.uk/pgmde/resources/howtoreflective.pdf

11 Royal College of General Practitioners. *RCGP Guide to the Revalidation of General Practitioners. Version 3*. London: Royal College of General Practitioners; 2010. www.rcgp.org.uk/_revalidation/revalidation_guide.aspx

12 Branch WT. Use of critical incident reports in medical education. *J Gen Intern Med*. 2005; **20**: 1063–7.

13 Bowie P, McKay J, Dalgetty E *et al*. A qualitative study of why general practitioners may participate in significant event analysis and educational peer assessment. *Qual Saf Health Care*. 2005; **14**: 185–9.

14 NHS Education for Scotland. *Significant Event Analysis*. www.nes.scot.nhs.uk/pharmacy/CPD/sea

15 Pringle M, Bradley CP, Carmichael CM *et al*. Significant event auditing. A study of the feasibility and potential of case-based auditing in primary medical care. *Occas Pap R Coll Gen Pract*. 1995; **70**: i–viii, 1–71.

FURTHER READING

- Bolton G. Write to learn: reflective practice writing. *InnovAiT*. 2009; **2**: 752–4.
- Chambers R, Wakley G. *Clinical Audit in Primary Care: demonstrating quality and outcomes*. Oxford: Radcliffe Publishing; 2005.
- Further information about the stages of self-directed learning (SSDL) model and other works can be found at www.longleaf.net/ggrow
- Gibbs G. *Learning by Doing: a guide to teaching and learning methods*. Cheltenham: Geography Discipline Network, University of Gloucestershire; 1988. www2.glos.ac.uk/gdn/gibbs/index.htm
- National Patient Safety Agency. www.npsa.nhs.uk
- Williams S. Dropping the baton. *Casebook*. 2010; **18**: 8–11. (Includes a discussion of the importance of handovers.)

CHAPTER 6

Developing your teaching style and techniques

This chapter will help you to understand your natural teaching style and consider how to adapt it to various learners' needs to help them progress from being dependent to self-directed learners. Just as the learner has a favoured learning style, you will have a preferred teaching style. Your teaching style has a powerful effect on the dynamics of their learning experience. Thus you should adapt it or adopt more appropriate styles according to the purpose of your teaching.

An effective teacher does not just impart knowledge and skills, but does so in a way that engages learners and leaves them with a deeper understanding and ability to interpret that freshly gained knowledge, or to apply those new skills. The effective teacher empowers a student to want to learn more, to actually do so and to put their learning into practice.

BE AWARE OF YOUR OWN TEACHING STYLE(S)

Your appearance, voice and what you say are vitally important in addition to your teaching style. Your gestures and body language should not be distracting, and should complement your voice and the messages of your teaching.

You will have developed your teaching style as a result of what comes naturally to you, the training and feedback that you have received, and your experience. There may have been some particular role models who have influenced your style, as you have unconsciously emulated teachers whom you have found inspiring, or deliberately avoided being like those with an off-putting style. You might have a quiet, introverted personality and tend towards the *all-round flexible and adaptable* teaching style, or you may be an extrovert and enjoy the *big conference* teaching style (see below). Your healthcare discipline may also influence your teaching style. Doctors often adopt a dominating style and expect to be in charge, whereas nurses and allied health professionals may be more learner-centred.

You will become more aware of the nature of the style that you are using and how effective it is from continuing reflection, feedback and evaluation of your teaching over the years. However, good performance requires a supportive teaching environment, sufficient time to deliver the required scope and level of learning, a reasonable teacher/

learner ratio and a good match between learners' needs and your expertise/knowledge. Non-work-related worries, such as health or financial concerns, working in unfamiliar settings or being generally harassed, may affect your performance and awareness of your teaching style. These factors may affect your concentration, restrict your intuitive powers and limit your reflective insights.

You may not feel comfortable using all teaching styles. However, your ability to vary your teaching style according to learners' needs and level(s) and the purpose of the learning activity will depend on your insight. Exploit those styles that you are good at, and practise the other styles for delivering learning when there is minimal pressure and you can obtain constructive feedback.

Investigate your teaching style

One way of considering the varied range of teaching styles is the Staffordshire Evaluation of Teaching Styles (SETS) approach.[1] The underpinning research determined six main styles.

1 **The all-round flexible and adaptable teacher** can use many different skills, can teach both peers and juniors, and is very aware of the whole environment both of teaching and of the learners.
2 **The student-centred, sensitive teacher** is very learner-centred, teaches in small groups, with emotions to the fore, using role play and drama, and is not comfortable doing straight presentations.
3 **The official formal curriculum teacher** is very well prepared, accredited, is very aware of and adheres to the formal curriculum, and follows external targets.
4 **The straight-facts, no-nonsense teacher** likes to teach the clear facts, with straight talking, concentrating on specific skills, and much prefers not to be involved with multi-professional teaching and learning.
5 **The big conference teacher** most enjoys standing up in front of a large audience, and does not like sitting in groups or one-to-one teaching.
6 **The one-off teacher** likes to deliver small self-contained topics, on a one-to-one basis, with no props to help and no follow-up.

Try working out your preferred teaching style(s) by completing the four steps of the next exercise:

➤ **Step 1.** Fill in the questionnaire.
➤ **Step 2.** Score your answers.
➤ **Step 3.** Rate each of the six teaching styles.
➤ **Step 4.** Plot your ratings to compare and contrast your preferences for each of the six teaching styles.

STEP 1: WORK OUT YOUR PREFERRED TEACHING STYLE(S) BY ANSWERING THE FOLLOWING QUESTIONS.

Rate the extent to which you agree with each of the statements below from 1 (do not agree at all) to 5 (very strongly agree).

	Do not agree at all				Very strongly agree
Q1. I vary my approach depending on my audience	1	2	3	4	5
Q2. I am less comfortable giving straight presentations than teaching through games and exercises	1	2	3	4	5
Q3. I prefer to teach through games to relay learning	1	2	3	4	5
Q4. I like having external targets to determine the course of learning	1	2	3	4	5
Q5. I prefer teaching sessions that are self-contained with no follow-up	1	2	3	4	5
Q6. Props often detract from a talk	1	2	3	4	5
Q7. I am comfortable addressing large audiences	1	2	3	4	5
Q8. Preparation for my teaching focuses on me and my role	1	2	3	4	5
Q9. I am usually standing up when I teach	1	2	3	4	5
Q10. The best teaching sessions convey straight facts in a clear way	1	2	3	4	5
Q11. I avoid being distracted from running sessions the way I plan to run them	1	2	3	4	5
Q12. I am happy teaching general skills	1	2	3	4	5
Q13. I put no value on being formally employed as a teacher	1	2	3	4	5
Q14. I dislike one-to-one (tutor) teaching	1	2	3	4	5
Q15. I am consistent in delivery of a topic, whatever the audience	1	2	3	4	5
Q16. I like to give students the opportunity to explore how to learn	1	2	3	4	5
Q17. I have developed my own style as a teacher	1	2	3	4	5
Q18. I prefer one-to-one (tutor) teaching	1	2	3	4	5
Q19. Eliciting emotions through role play or drama is a valuable aspect of teaching	1	2	3	4	5
Q20. I am comfortable using humour in my teaching	1	2	3	4	5
Q21. I am rarely sitting down when teaching students	1	2	3	4	5
Q22. It is important to me that my teaching is accredited by an official body	1	2	3	4	5
Q23. I am uncomfortable when I have multi-professional groups of learners to teach	1	2	3	4	5
Q24. I am at my best when organising my teaching to fit an external curriculum or organisational structure	1	2	3	4	5

STEP 2: COMPLETE YOUR SCORING GRID.

Write your score for each of the questions in the correct boxes, then add up the columns to obtain your score for each of the six teaching styles (out of a maximum of 20 marks).

Question	Style 1	Style 2	Style 3	Style 4	Style 5	Style 6
Q1	Q1 =					
Q2		Q2 =				
Q3		Q3 =				
Q4			Q4 =			
Q5						Q5 =
Q6						Q6 =
Q7					Q7 =	
Q8			Q8 =			
Q9					Q9 =	
Q10				Q10 =		
Q11				Q11 =		
Q12	Q12 =					
Q13						Q13 =
Q14					Q14 =	
Q15				Q15 =		
Q16		Q16 =				
Q17	Q17 =					
Q18						Q18 =
Q19		Q19 =				
Q20	Q20 =					
Q21					Q21 =	
Q22			Q22 =			
Q23				Q23 =		
Q24			Q24 =			
Totals						

STEP 3: RATE EACH TEACHING STYLE.

Fill in your scores, obtained from the chart totals in Step 2, in the six boxes against each of the teaching styles listed below.

		Your scores
Style 1	The all-round flexible and adaptable teacher	
Style 2	The student-centred, sensitive teacher	
Style 3	The official formal curriculum teacher	
Style 4	The straight-facts, no-nonsense teacher	
Style 5	The big conference teacher	
Style 6	The one-off teacher	

Now you have the six scores out of 20 for your self-evaluation of your preferred teaching styles.

STEP 4: PLOT YOUR PREFERRED TEACHING STYLE(S) ON THE SETS HEXAGON.

Plot the marks, from the rating sheet in Step 3, with a cross along each of the six axes to represent your score for each of the six teaching styles. Join up the crosses to produce a shape that represents your own combination of styles.

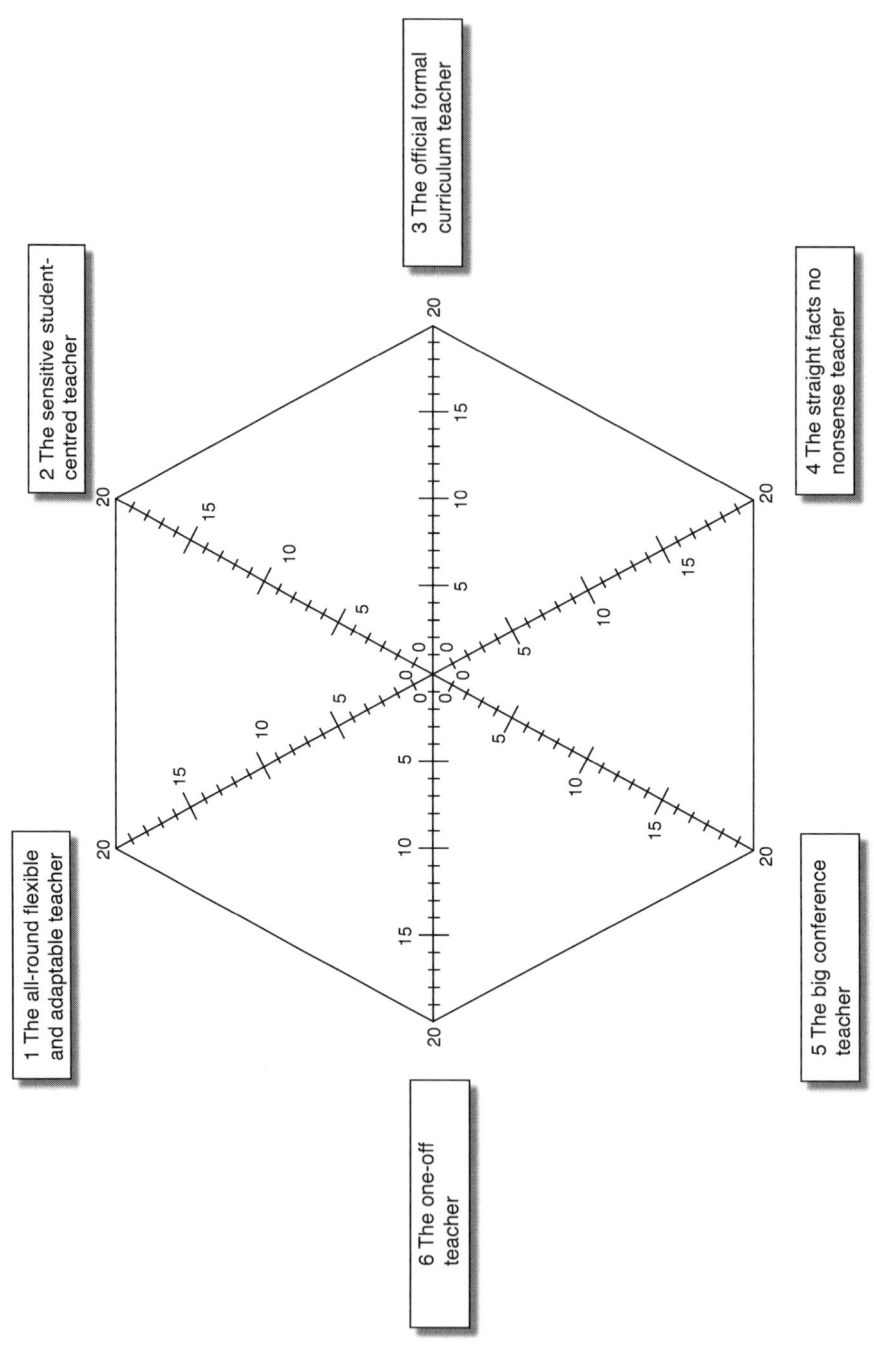

1 The all-round flexible and adaptable teacher

2 The sensitive student-centred teacher

3 The official formal curriculum teacher

4 The straight facts no nonsense teacher

5 The big conference teacher

6 The one-off teacher

TAILORING YOUR TEACHING STYLE(S) TO STUDENTS' LEARNING STYLE(S)

Consider whether your preferred teaching style suits the learning style(s) and needs of your learners for particular teaching episodes. If it does not, you should switch or adapt your teaching style to engage with your learners better and, hopefully, to improve their understanding, knowledge and skills. The main approaches to tailoring your teaching style to learners' needs are summarised below.

Matching

This will encourage learners to be interested and involved. Introverts prefer well-structured situations, so a *straight-facts, no-nonsense* teaching style might suit this type of learner. Extroverts prefer less structured situations, so the *all-round flexible and adaptable* teaching style should be suitable for these learners.

Allowing choice

The *all-round flexible and adaptable* teaching style should suit learners from a range of backgrounds and with various levels of knowledge and skills, as you vary your style and content to match their needs and preferences. You should guide them in an engaging way using your *sensitive, student-centred* style.

Providing several different methods of learning on the same course

If this approach is used, all of the learners should find something that suits them during the course, whether they are dependent, interested, involved or self-directed learners. The *all-round flexible and adaptable* teaching style fits well, as it motivates and guides interested and involved learners. The *sensitive, student-centred* teacher will craft their teaching to the various learning styles of a group of learners and the specific needs of individual learners, handling dependent learners as well as firing up self-directed learners. The *official curriculum* teaching style is more authoritarian, and will be useful for covering the formal content of a course required for accreditation. The *big conference* teaching style could be useful for providing variety to all kinds of learners, and a *one-off* teaching style might make the most of experts brought in as external speakers. The *straight-facts, no-nonsense* style could help during revision sessions for dependent learners or for students who are falling behind with their course work.

Independent study for self-directed learners

The *all-round flexible and adaptable* teacher will facilitate and encourage the freedom to study as independent learning, especially with more mature learners.

MATCHING YOUR TEACHING STYLE TO LEARNERS' NEEDS AND PREFERENCES

Another way of thinking about different teaching styles relates to your teaching *personality*. We shall return to Grow's stages of self-directed learning (SSDL) model with four types of delivery of teaching (*see* Chapter 5):[2,3]

➤ T1: authority; coach
➤ T2: motivator; guide
➤ T3: facilitator
➤ T4: consultant; delegator.

TABLE 6.1 Teaching delivery styles matched against the six SETS teaching styles

Teaching delivery	SETS teaching styles					
	All-round flexible	Student-centred	Official curriculum	Straight facts	Big conference	One-off
Authority	✓		✓	✓	✓	
Motivator	✓	✓	maybe		maybe	maybe
Facilitator	✓	✓				✓
Delegator	✓	✓				✓

You need various types of teaching delivery described in the SSDL model for the six teaching styles of the SETS model. Different ways of delivering teaching (authoritarian, motivational, facilitatory and delegator) can be applied to the six different SETS teaching styles and situations (*see* Table 6.1).

The SSDL model suggests why 'good teaching' is widely misunderstood. Often people think that there is only one way to teach well – and usually it is their way!

Awards generally go to teachers who are outstanding in one of the first two stages, either the one who provides copious structured information and instruction (sometimes called 'bucket filling', where the learner is seen as a vessel ready to be filled with information from the teacher) or the one who leads and motivates learners. Awards less often go to teachers who encourage learners to develop independently, or those who engage the most advanced learners with deep, open-ended problems.

'Good teaching' for one learner may not be 'good teaching' for another, or even for the same learner at a different stage of development. Good teaching does two things. It matches the learner's stage of self-direction, and it empowers the learner to progress towards greater self-direction. Good teaching is situational, yet it promotes the long-term development of the learner.

Mismatch between teaching style and stage of learning

Even if adult teachers recognise that adult learners are not all necessarily self-directed learners, it is widely assumed that adults will become self-directed after a few sessions of explaining the concept.

However, not all adults become self-directed just because they have been told to do so. Adult learners can be at any of the four learning stages, but the literature on adult education is dominated by advocates of what the SSDL model would call a Stage 3 method – a facilitative approach, emphasising group activity. However, teachers may sometimes need to approach certain learners in a directive, authoritarian style, and then gradually equip those learners with the skills, self-concept and motivation necessary to pursue learning in a more self-directed manner.

Advocates of a classroom in which learner and teacher receive equal respect acknowledge the paradoxical need to be directive, as Grow states:

> On the one hand, I cannot manipulate. On the other hand, I cannot leave the students by themselves. The opposite of these two possibilities is being radically

democratic. That means accepting the directive nature of education. There is a directiveness in education which never allows it to be neutral. My role is not to be silent.[2]

Every stage involves balancing the teacher's power with the learner's emerging self-direction.

The temptations of each teaching style

The temptation for the Stage 1 teacher is to be authoritarian in a punitive, controlling way that stifles initiative and creates resistance and dependency.

The temptation for the Stage 2 teacher is to remain on centre stage, inspiring all who will listen but leaving them with no more learning skills or self-motivation than when they started.

The Stage 3 teacher can disappear into the group and demoralise learners by 'accepting and valuing almost anything from anybody.'

The Stage 4 teacher can withdraw too much from the learning experience, lose touch, fail to monitor progress, and let learners hang themselves with rope they are not yet accustomed to handling.

In each instance, the teacher may falter in the immensely difficult juggling act of becoming 'vitally, vigorously, creatively, energetically, and inspiringly unnecessary.'

Recursive teaching

The SSDL model describes a progression of stages, but the progress of a learner or class will rarely be linear, and most classes will contain learners at different stages of self-direction. A more realistic version of the model would be non-linear and iterative.

Consider a course designed according to the Stage 3 model. The teacher serves as group facilitator, with the job of empowering learners to take greater charge of their learning and making certain that they master advanced levels of the subject matter. Most of the work takes place in the Stage 3 arena, where the teacher attempts to phase out external leadership and empower more self-direction.

However, there will be times when other learning modes are necessary. When the group (or some of its members) are deficient in basic skills, they may require drill and practice, a Stage 1 approach. (Even advanced learners sometimes choose T1 teachers who push them to achieve goals that they cannot achieve under their own motivation.) Sometimes the T3 teacher may determine that coaching or confrontation is necessary to reach a learner. The class may loop back to the Stage 1 mode for a while before returning to Stage 3.

Continued motivation and encouragement may sometimes be supplied by members of the class, but it may require the teacher to shift to the Stage 2 mode and provide it.

At times the teacher's knowledge matters more than anything else; lecturing may be the best possible response at that point. During the lecture, the class loops back to the Stage 1 or Stage 2 mode, and then returns to the group interaction and subtle facilitation of the Stage 3 mode.

When individuals or subgroups become ready to exert self-direction and leadership, these learners can go into the S4 mode, independently carry out a project and then come back to the group and teach the results. With the Stage 3 facilitated mode of teaching as a base, the class can loop out to the other three stages when appropriate.

Tips from experienced teachers

- Don't become lazy. Continue to adapt your teaching style for your learners, and put their needs first.
- Specify the requirements for an assignment in a supportive way so that dependent learners can more easily progress to being self-directed as they plan and apply their newly acquired knowledge and skills.
- Stay humble. Welcome all feedback from learners (especially that which you could not have predicted), and continue to reflect on how you might improve your future delivery of teaching to different groups of learners.
- Listen, listen, listen . . . to your learners.

A class that is focused on any stage of learning from S1 to S4 can draw support from the earlier stages and lean towards the later stages. Many courses centre around a series of Stage 1/Stage 2 lectures, but have a weekly discussion group that is more in the Stage 3 mode. 'Looping' may be a more effective way to use the SSDL concept than trying to follow a sequence of linear stages.

REFERENCES

1 Mohanna K, Chambers R, Wall D. *Your Teaching Style; a practical guide to understanding, developing and improving.* Oxford: Radcliffe Publishing; 2008.
2 Grow GP. Teaching learners to be self-directed. *Adult Educ Quarterly.* 1996; **41:** 125–49.
3 www.longleaf.net/ggrow

FURTHER READING

- Bennett SN. *Teaching Styles and Pupil Progress.* London: Open Books; 1976.
- Butler KA. *Learning and Teaching Style: in theory and practice.* Columbia, CT: The Learner's Dimension; 1984.
- Entwistle NJ. *Styles of Learning and Teaching.* London: David Fulton Publishers; 1988.
- Kaufman DM, Mann KV, Jennett PA. *Teaching and Learning in Medical Education: how theory can inform practice.* Edinburgh: Association for the Study of Medical Education; 2000.

CHAPTER 7

Curriculum: constructing a programme for learning

Mike Deighan

This chapter offers a practical approach to planning a course of study for individuals or groups of learners.

WHAT IS CURRICULUM?

Recently, the term 'curriculum' has come to mean a document produced by a national body and handed down. For example, since the creation of the Postgraduate Medical Education and Training Board (PMETB), medical education in the UK has seen a flurry of activity within the Medical Royal Colleges, producing national curricula.

The term 'curriculum' is also used to refer to what teachers do – that is, plan, implement and evaluate their educational programmes. Until the advent of the National Curriculum for Schools,[1] this planning and implementation cycle was what was meant by curriculum. In UK nursing and undergraduate medicine, curricula are still conceived at school level.

There is a certain tension between older and current meanings, so check what is meant whenever the word 'curriculum' is used. Some authors use the term *curriculum design* to refer to official processes, and the term *curriculum development* to describe what teachers do. Both meanings are practically important for course planners, because the presence of a national curriculum usually means that a large amount of control over planning, content and assessment has passed from a local level to a higher authority. Whether this is a good thing depends upon the quality of the official document and the values of the teacher.

PLANNING A COURSE

For many who see curriculum as a simple matter of fitting content into a timetable, this section may seem unnecessary. There is insufficient space here to rehearse the arguments for a more complex view of curriculum planning (these can be found in Chapter 3 of Fish and Coles),[2] but the main justification hinges on the distinction between training and education:

> Education . . . deals with unknown outcomes, and circumstances which require a complex synthesis of knowledge, skills and experience to solve problems.

Education refers its questions and actions to principles and values rather than merely standards and criteria ... training ... has application when: a) there is some identifiable performance and/or skill that has to be mastered; and b) practice is required for the mastery of it. ... Effective learning in medical education ... includes elements of training set in the context of lifelong learning.[3]

The nature of professional knowledge and learning is covered elsewhere.[2,4–9] Essentially, practitioners learn from their professional practice in order to make the transition from novice to expert (*see* Box 7.1).

BOX 7.1 Progression from novice to expert (adapted from Eraut,[10] after Dreyfus)

Level 1: Novice

Rigid adherence to taught rules or plans

Little situational perception

No discretionary judgement

Level 2: Advanced beginner

Guidelines for action based on attributes or aspects (aspects are global characteristics of situations recognisable only after some prior experience)

Situational perception still limited

All attributes and aspects are treated separately and given equal importance

Level 3: Competent

Coping with crowdedness (the number of patients, activities, pieces of information, etc. competing for the individual's attention)

Now sees actions at least partially in terms of longer-term goals

Conscious deliberate planning

Standardised and routinised procedures

Level 4: Proficient

Sees situations holistically rather than in terms of aspects

Sees what is most important in a situation

Perceives deviations from the normal pattern

Decision making is less laboured

Uses maxims for guidance, whose meaning varies according to the situation

Level 5: Expert

No longer relies on rules, guidelines or maxims

Intuitive grasp of situations based on deep tacit understanding

Analytical approaches used only in novel situations, when problems occur or when justifying conclusions

Has a vision of what is possible

A large proportion of the knowledge that healthcare professionals use is implicit or tacit. This 'action knowledge'[10] is quicker and more intuitive, making it more useful than explicit knowledge, which would be slow and cumbersome in many clinical situations. A curriculum that puts the emphasis on the teaching and assessment of factual knowledge can have an adverse effect on the learning of less tangible professional qualities, such as creativity, imagination, enquiry, values and attitudes.[11]

How should I start to plan my course?

First, identify the broad aims of the course. Clarity will help subsequent course design and also explanation of the course to stakeholders. The more clearly learners understand your intentions, the greater will be their ability to take control of their own learning.

After deciding on the big picture, chunk down these aims into a medium-level course outline. This will depend on the decisions that you make on content, so concept mapping[12-14] may be helpful here.

As well as designing blocks of content, identify one or two themes that run through the whole course or through several elements. This gives unity to the course, allows learners to appreciate the interconnectedness of items, and breaks down barriers and undermines fixed perspectives. An alternative approach to linear curriculum planning is the concept of a spiral curriculum.[15,16] This addresses the lack of integration within healthcare education, and involves revisiting topics and subject areas over time.

Once you have a broad outline, think about course objectives (*see* Box 7.2). These are more specific than aims.

BOX 7.2 Clarifying curriculum objectives[17]

Step 1   Decide what kind of knowledge is to be involved

Step 2   Select the topics to teach

Step 3   Decide the purpose of teaching the topic and hence the level of knowledge that it is desirable for learners to acquire

Step 4   Put the package of objectives together and relate them to assessment tasks

---

After the curriculum objectives have been finalised, you can write schemes of work. Following these, the final units of design are individual lesson plans. These will depend on local circumstances and your own preferences.

The questions in Box 7.3 highlight the choices to be made in setting course aims and objectives.

BOX 7.3 Question 1: What is the context within which you are planning?

Is there a 'handed down' curriculum that you need to take into account?
Are you planning part of a larger curriculum and need to take account of other educators?
Are you free to make your own decisions?
Are there resource issues?

CONTEXT
Early decisions in curriculum planning
Curriculum planning rarely starts with a blank sheet of paper. You should be prepared for other educational activity, such as a written curriculum, a previous curriculum or examination syllabus, or other departments with which you may have to compete for the learner's attention.

If there is a national curriculum, you must first decide what purpose it serves for you.

If you have a 'handed down' curriculum (*see* Box 7.4), power resides in a higher authority. The other two options see power being exercised locally or even shared by the learner.

BOX 7.4 What is your attitude to a 'handed down' curriculum?

- It is a blueprint (from which we intend to make replicas).
- It is like a play (as directors, we follow the text but interpret it in our own way).
- It is like a springboard (a point of departure from which teachers and learners launch themselves).

Teachers can decide between two basic positions. One position cedes all authority to the national document for content, planning and assessment (*see* Figure 7.1), and the curriculum is used as a blueprint. In the other, the national curriculum is used as an authoritative resource, but teachers maintain their own judgement about suitable content and methods. Teachers may also want to retain a say in evaluation (*see* Figure 7.2).

This decision will depend on many factors, such as the quality of the national curriculum, the wishes of the learners, the wishes of teachers and the resources available.

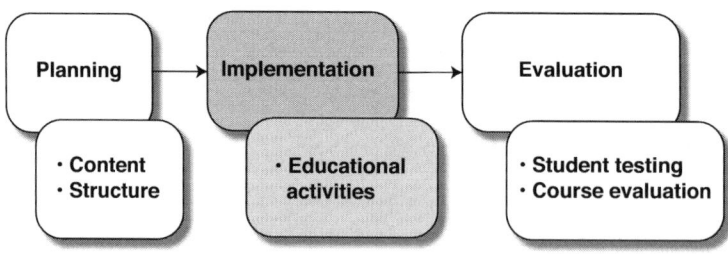

FIGURE 7.1

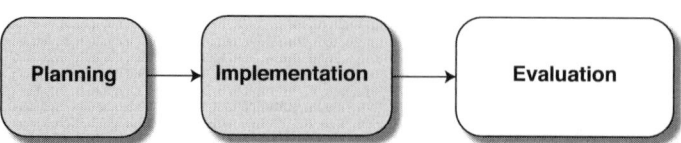

FIGURE 7.2

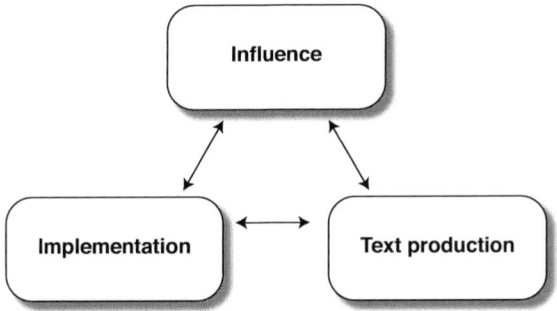

FIGURE 7.3

Designing a curriculum from scratch

If you get the opportunity to design a curriculum from scratch, don't waste it. Bowes et al.[18] have identified three areas of activity in the production of a curriculum, each of which plays a part in creating the success of the end product (*see* Figure 7.3).

If you are a curriculum writer, responsible for producing the text, be aware of the requirements of regulators (e.g. government, regulatory organisations) and other out-side bodies (e.g. professional organisations, student bodies, pressure groups).

The burden of history

Another context problem that faces curriculum writers is the burden of history. Both teachers and learners will often be attached to familiar content, teaching methods and assessments. The management of change is covered in Chapter 20, and that involved in introducing a curriculum is covered in Leach.[19]

CONTENT

There are many methods of determining content (*see* Box 7.5), including the Delphi technique (expert panel), critical incident survey (educational lessons of good and bad practice), task analysis (observation of practitioners), epidemiology (mortality and morbidity rates) and gap analysis (identifying what is missing from current practice).[20]

BOX 7.5 Question 2: How will you decide on the content of your curriculum?

What do you want learners to know?
What skills do they need to acquire?
What functions do you want learners to be able to perform by the end of the course?

Topics to include are those that:
➤ directly contribute to course objectives
➤ are essential building blocks to understanding later learning
➤ develop intellectual abilities such as critical thinking[21]
➤ make connections between elements of the curriculum.[21]

Content specification can be difficult. Although most learners and teachers are satisfied with broad brushstrokes, some want everything to be specified in detail. Such hyper-specification will result in a vast curriculum document that no one will read.[22] Another disadvantage of a detailed syllabus is that it often produces the demand that there shall be no teaching or assessment of anything that is not written into the curriculum. Given the rapid rate of change in the world of healthcare, you need to be able to incorporate new developments in healthcare professionals' training.

Structuring your content description

Traditionally, medical curricula were based on catalogues of diseases mapped on to body systems. Today, this biomedical, pathology-based approach is being abandoned in favour of a classification that addresses the relationship between the patient and the healthcare professional, and takes into account a more holistic understanding of the patient's world.

Swanson[23] distinguished between 'discipline' or 'organ systems' curricula and those that used a problem-based approach to learning. Today, the organisational structures of curricula take into account the relationship between healthcare professionals and society. Issues such as ethics, trust, accountability, healthcare professionals' self-awareness, their relationships with colleagues, the nature of healthcare services, health economics and leadership are often grouped under the term 'professionalism'. Examples of these can be found in 'The Five-Star Doctor',[24] ACGME,[19] PRISMS,[25] CanMEDS,[26] the Sheffield undergraduate curriculum[27,28] and generic postgraduate competences.[29]

Knowledge and understanding

Healthcare workers often overvalue factual knowledge, and this can have a distorting effect on curriculum planning. Biggs[17] defines various forms of knowledge:
➤ declarative knowledge:
 — knowing about things
 — knowledge that we can declare to someone in writing or verbally
➤ functioning knowledge:
 — knowledge that we put to work in problem solving, analysing or designing something, or in making an argument.

Functioning knowledge depends not only on knowing *facts* (declarative knowledge), but also on knowledge of *how* (procedural knowledge) and *when* and *why* (conditional knowledge). In total, 14 different types of knowledge have been defined.[30]

Another useful distinction is between academic and professional knowledge (*see* Table 7.1).

TABLE 7.1 Distinction between professional and academic knowledge (adapted from Biggs,[17] after Leinhardt[31])

Professional knowledge	Academic knowledge
Functioning, specific and pragmatic	Declarative, abstract and conceptual
Deals with executing, applying and making priorities	Deals with labelling, differentiating, elaborating and justifying

Tension arises between the knowledge of the 'ivory towers' of academia and the practice-bound practical 'know-how' of the professional, not only in the content but also in the way that knowledge is used. Learners can have problems transferring knowledge from abstract, academic discourse to real-world problems.[31]

Established, expert practitioners cannot always explain their decision-making processes. Their knowledge is unconscious, intuitive or tacit.

Learner-perceived needs and stakeholder needs

Learning needs assessment has clear gains, not least the avoidance of teaching people what they already know. However, a major disadvantage is that it can allow learners to limit their learning to what they are interested in, rather than what they need to know.

At the curriculum level, you should define what needs to be known and highlight the relative importance of each topic area, rather than solely focusing on learning gaps. When teaching, emphasise aspects that are usually poorly understood. With the shift towards self-directed learning,[32-34] learners often decide which events to attend in order to achieve their learning aims. Clear statements of intended outcomes help the learner with this.

Breadth and depth

Decide whether to cover all possible content superficially or selected topics in depth. Remember that 'the greatest enemy of understanding is coverage.'[17] Course planners must be prepared to omit enough topics to create the space needed to do justice to key areas.

Curriculum mapping

Curriculum mapping can clarify thinking in planning and in explaining a curriculum to learners and faculty. Harden[13] has provided examples of categories (*see* Figure 7.4).

ASSESSMENT

Traditionally, assessment and course evaluation occur at the end of the course. The argument for this has been that learning continues throughout the course and is expected to be maximal at the end.

Deeper analysis of the nature of professional learning[5,35,36] indicates that although knowledge is important, it is not sufficient for the kind of complex decisions that professionals need to make.

Beyond knowledge testing: Miller's pyramid (*see* Figure 7.5)

Knowledge testing is beloved by psychometricians, as candidates' scores remain fairly constant over time, and it is thus the best predictor of success. This makes it a strongly desirable feature of selection processes. However, it is overvalued for end-point assessment. Knowledge of something does not directly translate into capability.

Tate noted that during an oral examination, learners frequently demonstrate a high degree of knowledge about patient-centred consulting. However, when a video examination of consulting was introduced, actual application of this knowledge into patient-centred behaviour was extremely rare.[37]

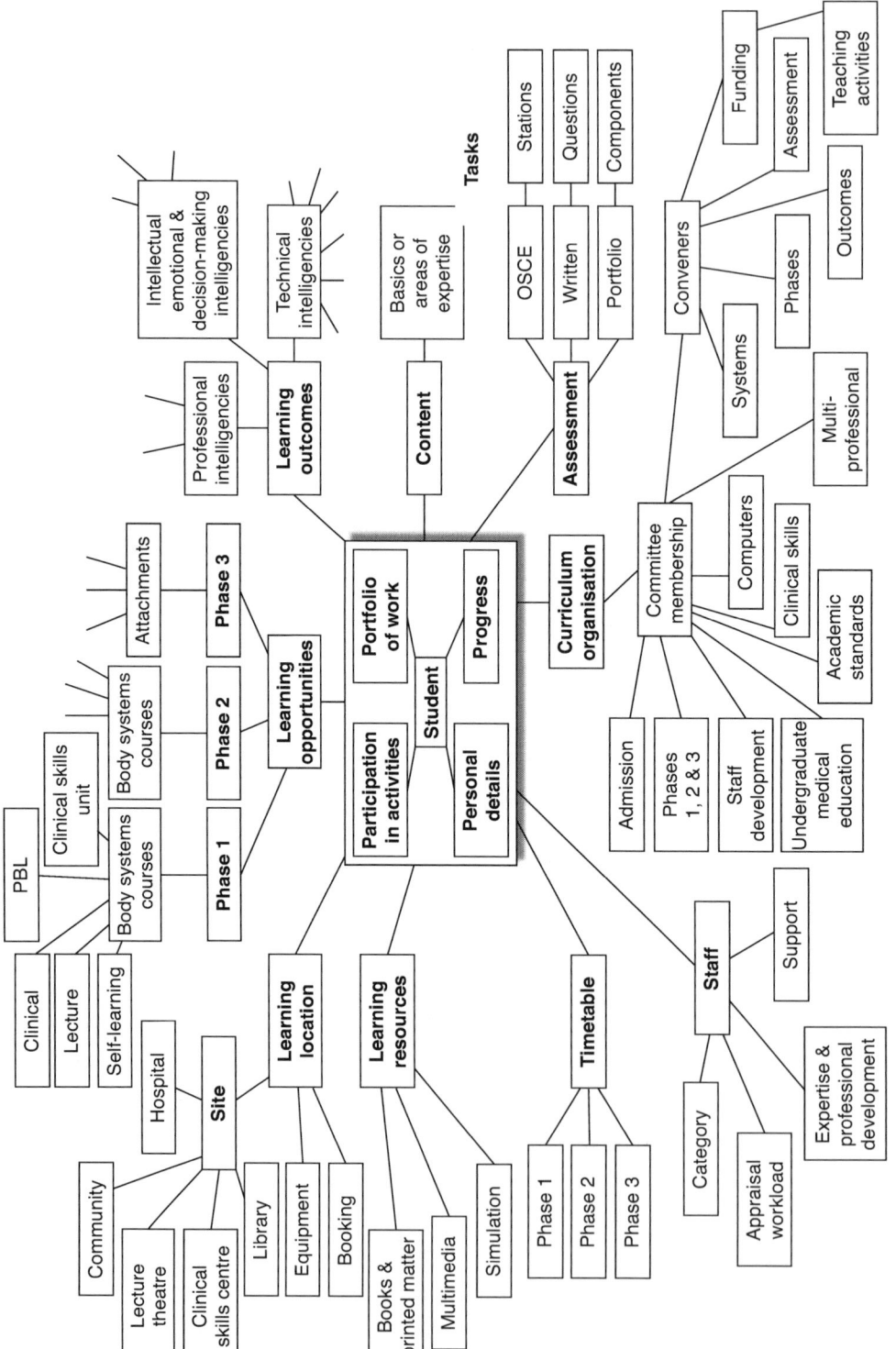

FIGURE 7.4

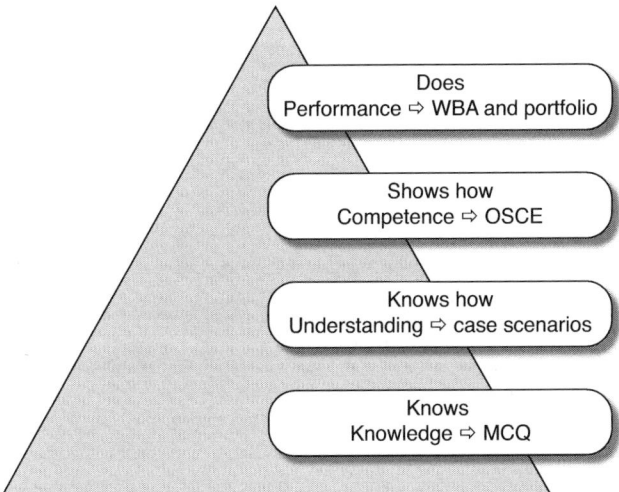

FIGURE 7.5

Miller argues that although knowledge is an important foundation for learning, professional assessments require methods that assess the application of knowledge to real-life situations and those in which the healthcare professional can demonstrate competence at complex tasks. Although testing competence is a useful assessment of learning, learners can demonstrate competence in examination situations by exhibiting behaviours that they do not use in real life.

The strongest educational argument for assessment over time is that, unlike competence, performance can only be measured over time.

Aligning curriculum and assessment

Aligning the curriculum with assessments is very important, not least because learners will be dissatisfied if they are not taught what they are assessed on. If you have control over assessment, this is much easier. However, assessment methods may be chosen without reference to the curriculum, pre-date the curriculum or be chosen by a different body of people. Fitting a curriculum to assessments is a common problem for teachers.

If curriculum items are not tested in a formal assessment, they are likely to be unpopular among (or ignored by) learners. Figures 7.6 and 7.7 illustrate this point – the teacher identifies learning objectives and creates learning opportunities for these objectives to be achieved. The learner, on the other hand, is more likely to first look at the assessments and then, from the same learning opportunities, achieve some of the objectives that the teacher set.[17] Unless the curriculum and the assessments are perfectly aligned, the learning that is achieved will be a subset of the original intended learning outcomes.

Should the curriculum sacrifice important or desirable aspects of education just to achieve good alignment with assessments? Consider the reality of life after the course. If there are important things that cannot be tested but which are essential for the learner to have mastered, then they must be included in the curriculum. Curriculum and assessments should align with the needs of the learner after the course (*see* Figure 7.8).

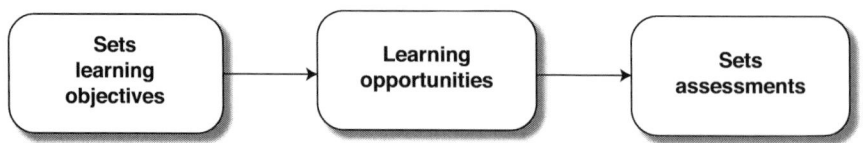

FIGURE 7.6

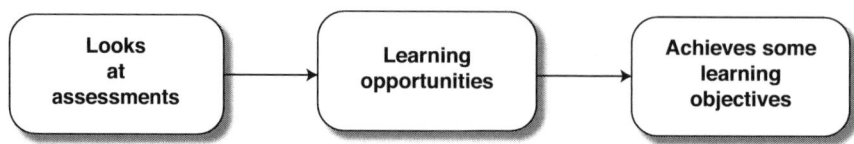

FIGURE 7.7

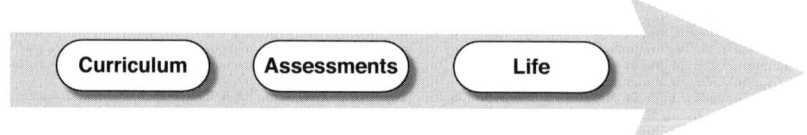

FIGURE 7.8

Choosing modes of assessment

Assessments are hugely important in improving learning, but this fact is often ignored in the education of healthcare professionals, where the emphasis is often on high-stakes assessment, which has little positive effect and many adverse effects on learning. Biggs has highlighted assessments which provide useful information to the course planner about what is being learned (*see* Table 7.2).[17]

ACTIVITIES

Activities have more uses than just delivering content. They can be important in motivating learners, conveying attitudes or getting learners to respond to curricular content. Be careful to place the focus of activities on those that the learners need, rather than those that you need to use to teach.

The classroom and the workplace

Much has been written about the poor quality of clinical teaching,[38–40] and this may be why many learners prefer learning on courses rather than in the workplace. Learners also prefer things to be black and white, rather than the various shades of grey of real-life events. Eraut[41] has highlighted the richness of the workplace for learning (*see* Table 7.3 and Chapter 5).

TABLE 7.2 Assessments and their uses (adapted from Biggs[17])

	Assessment mode	Most likely kind of learning assessed
Extended prose, essay type	Essay exam	Rote, question spotting, speed structuring
	Open book	As above but less memory, coverage
	Assignment, take-home	Read widely, interrelate, organise, apply, copy
Objective test	Multiple choice	Recognition, strategy, comprehension
	Ordered outcome	Hierarchies of understanding
Performance assessment	Practicum	Skills needed in real life
	Seminar, presentation	Communication skills
	Posters	Concentrating on relevance, application
	Interviewing	Responding interactively
	Critical incidents	Reflection, application, sense of relevance
	Project	Research skills
	Reflective journal	Reflection, application, sense of relevance
	Case study, problems	Application, professional skills
	Portfolio	Reflection, creativity, unintended outcomes
Rapid assessments (large class)	Concept maps	Coverage, relationships
	Venn diagrams	Relationships
	Three-minute essay	Level of understanding, sense of relevance
	Gobbets	Realising the importance of significant detail
	Short answer	Recall units of information, coverage
	Letter-to-a-friend	Holistic understanding, application, reflection
	Cloze test (passages of text with missing words to be completed)	Comprehension of main ideas

TABLE 7.3 Learning in the workplace

Work processes with learning as a by-product	Learning activities located within work or learning processes	Learning processes at or near the workplace
Participation in group processes	Asking questions	Being supervised
Working alongside others	Listening	Being coached
Consultation	Observing	Being mentored
Tackling challenging tasks and roles	Obtaining information	Shadowing
Problem solving	Learning from mistakes	Visiting other sites
Trying things out	Reflecting	Independent study
Working with patients	Locating resource people	Conferences
	Giving and receiving feedback	Short courses
		Working for a qualification

TABLE 7.4 Essential and ideal features of activities[42]

Essential features	Ideal features
Built around key curriculum ideas	Motivational
Feasible and cost-effective	Address multiple goals
Time and resource efficient	Topic currency related to what is current or recently taught or experienced
Pitched at the right level	
Challenging – encourage higher-order thinking (e.g. analysis, interpretation, synthesis)	Related to real world
	Connect declarative knowledge (know *that*) with procedural knowledge (know *how*)
Not frustrating	Encourage self-directedness

Which activities are effective?

Aligning activities with your curriculum aims is essential (*see* Table 7.4). (*See* Chapter 8 for further information on *matching methods with message*.)

INSIGHTS FROM CURRICULUM THEORY
Much of what is learned is not in the curriculum

Hafferty[43] delineates two useful categories beyond 'the stated, intended, formally offered and endorsed curriculum':

1 the **informal curriculum** – the unscripted, highly interpersonal ad-hoc teaching
2 the **hidden curriculum** – the 'set of influences that function at the level of organisational structure and culture.'

Both of these categories of unstated aims have beneficial and adverse effects.

Teachers often assume a causal relationship between teaching and learning. However, much of what is learned is not taught. Even when what is learned is what you intended, it may not be learned from you. Learners may use sources other than your teaching for their knowledge. Sadly, even though learners don't always learn what is intended, they often learn lessons that teachers would not intend or might reject. The hidden curriculum is potent.[44] Your behaviour is the model upon which your learners base theirs.

The 'hidden curriculum'[45] describes the implicit way in which social norms are conveyed by academic institutions – the unofficial expectations relating to social attitudes and behaviours. For example, the hidden curriculum has been used to explain how, contrary to the expressed intention of the curriculum, medical students can be socialised by the prevailing culture into treating patients as objects:

> Today's medical care, while being technologically advanced, is experienced by many patients as impersonal and dehumanizing. Medical schools have responded by trying to teach the human dimensions of care. These efforts, however, are often thwarted by the culture of medicine, which places a premium on technology at the expense of interpersonal relationships.[46]

Hodges describes how some authors see the selection and recruitment of faculty staff as being 'aimed as much at the economic control of the profession as at social advancement.'[47]

Learners are aware of the hidden curriculum,[48] and they know that it has a profound effect on their learning, but its lessons can be unclear to them. They often associate facts with the formal curriculum, and 'learning how to be a doctor' with the hidden curriculum. Hidden lessons on behaviour are often worked out through oral and written narratives, such as the story in Box 7.6.[49]

BOX 7.6 An error of omission[49]

The patient, an elderly lady, was blind and deaf without speech. She had been brought in as an emergency case, clutching her abdomen and moaning. She had been like that for a couple of hours, and had also vomited several times. On examination she had some epigastric tenderness, her heart and lungs were normal, and her blood pressure was slightly low. Routine investigations were ordered; a drip was set up, and the team moved on.

On the next round the patient was still in severe pain. Nothing new had turned up. Her serum haemoglobin concentration, blood biochemistry, and chest and abdominal radiographs were normal. We hesitated over whether to provide pain relief. Antispasmodic drugs had been ineffective. An ultrasound scan ruled out problems with the patient's gallbladder. Endoscopy took another day to organise and produced negative results. The patient's pain and sickness continued. On the fifth day she died, with the causes undiagnosed, and her suffering unrelieved.

As house officer on the ward I had to prepare a case summary. Fishing in the pack of X-ray films for the reports I caught the long strip of an electrocardiogram. It bore the date of admission. I had asked a nurse to do it as part of the routine work-up, but had not remembered to check the results. The textbook signs of an extensive acute myocardial infarction were plain even to my untrained eye.

> I took the tracing to the senior consultant's office. He cast a glance over it and then stared at me for two uncomfortably long seconds.
>
> 'Making a fuss about this won't bring her back', he said. He tore off the old date and then in a firm hand wrote the current date under the patient's name.
>
> 'She has died of an acute myocardial infarction. *But let this be a lesson to all of us.*'

How should a curriculum or course writer manage an informal and hidden curriculum?

Can these two concepts be of any use to the planner given that, by definition, they are outside what is intended and stated? There are two ways in which the planner should anticipate informal and hidden elements in the curriculum, even though neither will be entirely predictable or under their control. The informal curriculum offers opportunities to develop learning in unplanned but beneficial ways if generic guidance is given.

The hidden curriculum is difficult to predict or influence, but transmission of social values is likely, so should be anticipated and influenced in a positive way.

Importance of case studies and narratives

Stories can be powerful learning tools.[50] Build them into your courses to help learners to become aware of hidden aspects of their work. Benner[51] advocates the use of case studies in teaching.

Learning occurs when stories and experiences are interweaved with knowledge and theory. According to Benner:

> Currently, the language used to talk about nursing practice is too simple, formal, and context-free to capture the essence and complexity of expert nursing . . . experience is not the mere passage of time or longevity; it is the refinement of preconceived notions and theory by encountering many actual practical situations that add nuances or shades of differences to theory.[51]

The importance of emotional involvement in this process is emphasised:

> . . . unless the trainee stays emotionally involved and accepts the joy of a job well done, as well as the remorse of mistakes, [they] will not develop further, and will eventually burn out trying to keep track of all the features and aspects, rules and maxims that modern medicine requires. In general, resistance to involvement and risk leads to stagnation and ultimately to boredom and regression.[52]

Importance of values

Some curricula are written without reference to values, yet in the end it is the values that the curriculum expresses and how they relate to the values of teachers and learners that will determine the success of the curriculum. If the values expressed in the curriculum are not in line with those of the faculty who deliver the teaching, the curriculum will fail.

CHOOSING FROM THE MANY OPTIONS: WHAT PRODUCT AM I AIMING FOR?

Education can be seen as a product, a process, research or discovery (*see* Table 7.5).

TABLE 7.5 Three approaches to education and their effect on curriculum design (adapted from Fish and Coles[2])

	Education as a product	Education as a process	Education as research
Intention	Teacher transmits knowledge	Teacher promotes knowledge	Learners explore understanding
Locus of knowledge	Teacher	Teachers and learners	Learner group
Student activities	Passive learners	Active learners	Aware of selves as active learners and negotiators
Motivation via	Teacher	Own active learning	Group learning and active learning
Sees learner as	Receiver of knowledge	Active seeker of knowledge	Discoverer or reconstructor of own knowledge
Sees teacher as	Teller Instructor	Seeker Catalyst	Facilitator Neutral chair
Teaching activities	Lecturing	Facilitates learning Sets up problems Probably knows answers	Teacher is leader within group but learns alongside them
Sees assessment as	End-of-course tests Summative teacher assessment	Part of teaching Part of learning Formative – and summative	Self-assessment Group assessment Aiding understanding
Plans by means of	Aims, objectives, detailed method for whole session, summative assessment	Aims, intentions, principles of procedure, list of content, assessment as part of this process	Aims, intentions, a negotiated agenda, counselling-type methods, assessment within this process
View of professional	Teacher is a performer whose performance is significant in the quality of the learner's education	Teacher is a facilitator who sets up learning for learners, and whose input features less in the sessions	Teacher is a facilitator who learns alongside learners, but this can only be on a highly disciplined basis

When planning a course, you can choose between these three perspectives while being mindful of what kind of healthcare professional is needed. Remember the distinction between training and education:[53]

> Training . . . prepares the learner to perform tasks already identified and described, by methods which have gained general approval. . . . Education teaches us to solve problems, the nature of which may not be known at the time when the education is taking place, and the solutions to which cannot be seen or even imagined by the teachers.[53]

CONCLUSION

Evaluation of your curriculum will depend on the model of curriculum you proposed. If you are using the product version, evaluation will be by means of a questionnaire designed by you, and will be answered anonymously to ensure that it does not affect the assessments. If you see education as a process, there may be a discussion among learners and teachers about what worked and what did not work, in order to develop an outline for next time. Those who see curriculum as research will not use evaluation, because they assess their experience throughout the course and change the content and methods to suit their needs. They will point out to you that evaluation at the end of a course is only a snapshot reaction to recent events, and they will only find out how good it has been in the months and years ahead.

An external view is often helpful, but differences of opinion are to be expected:

> In education, interpretation is central and interpretations can be in contention with each other, so that deliberation is not merely inevitable but rather is essential. Rather than being a weakness of educational thinking, this is one of its supreme strengths, especially for curriculum development, where discussion that focuses on the diversity of views about educational values is a key way of arriving at a shared understanding of what ought to happen for the best, and how this may be achieved.[2]

These sentiments are echoed by Young:

> A curriculum is always a contested concept which links ideas about knowledge and learning to an implicit or explicit set of educational purposes and goals for society.[54]

Tips from experienced teachers

- Planning a course (curriculum) involves blending content with timetable.[55]
- When dealing with a 'handed down' curriculum, you should make decisions on structuring and what to emphasise or omit.
- Curriculum decisions can be problematic, and choices may depend on your values.
- When planning education, consider what view of learning you wish to promote.
- Professional knowledge is complex and cannot be transmitted as a product. Education is distinct from training.
- Healthcare professionals need to make creative decisions. To be effective, their learning must be based on their practice.
- You must understand the relationship between theory and practice.
- Look beyond the course to the world that learners will be entering, and create learning outcomes that are relevant to life outside the classroom.

REFERENCES

1 Office of Public Sector Information. *Education Reform Act*. London: HMSO; 1988.
2 Fish D, Coles C. *Medical Education: developing a curriculum for practice*. Maidenhead: Open University Press; 2005.
3 Brigden DN, Grieveson B. Lifelong learning. *Prim Dental Care*. 2003; **10**: 31–2.
4 Schön DA. *The Reflective Practitioner: how professionals think in action*. New York: Basic Books; 1983.
5 Eraut M. *Developing Professional Knowledge and Competence*. London: RoutledgeFalmer; 1994.
6 Berragan L. Nursing practice draws upon several different ways of knowing. *J Clin Nurs*. 1998; **7**: 209–17.
7 Elstein AS, Bordage G. Psychology of clinical reasoning. In: Dowie J, Elstein A, eds. *Professional Judgement: a reader in clinical decision making*. Cambridge: Cambridge University Press; 1991.
8 Regehr G, Norman GR. Issues in cognitive psychology: implications for professional education. *Acad Med*. 1996; **71**: 988–1001.
9 Atkinson T, Claxton G. *The Intuitive Practitioner: on the value of not always knowing what one is doing*. Buckingham: Open University Press; 2000.
10 Eraut M. Non-formal learning and tacit knowledge in professional work. *Br J Educ Psychol*. 2000; **70**: 113–36.
11 Curtis R, Weeden P, Winter J. Measurement, judgement, criteria and expertise. In: Atkinson T, Claxton G, eds. *The Intuitive Practitioner: on the value of not always knowing what one is doing*. Buckingham: Open University Press; 2000. pp. 220–38.
12 Watson GR. What is . . . concept mapping? *Med Teacher*. 1989; **11**: 265–9.
13 Harden RM. AMEE Guide No. 21: Curriculum mapping: a tool for transparent and authentic teaching and learning. *Med Teacher*. 2001; **23**: 123–37.
14 Novak JD, Cañas AJ. *The Theory Underlying Concept Maps and How to Construct and Use Them*. Pensacola, FL: Florida Institute for Human and Machine Cognition; 2008.
15 Bruner JS. *The Process of Education*: Cambridge, MA: Harvard University Press; 1960.
16 Harden RM, Stamper N. What is a spiral curriculum? *Med Teacher*. 1999; **21**: 141–3.

17 Biggs JB. *Teaching for Quality Learning at University: what the student does.* Maidenhead: Society for Research into Higher Education and Open University Press; 2003.

18 Bowe R, Ball SJ, Gold A. *Reforming Education and Changing Schools: case studies in policy sociology.* London: Routledge; 1992.

19 Leach DC. Changing education to improve patient care. *Qual Health Care.* 2001; **10** (Suppl. 2): ii54–8.

20 Dunn WR, Hamilton DD, Harden RM. Techniques of identifying competencies needed of doctors. *Med Teacher.* 1985; **7**: 15–25.

21 Harden RM. Ten questions to ask when planning a course or curriculum. *Med Educ.* 1986; **20**: 356–65.

22 Batalden P, Leach D, Swing S *et al.* General competencies and accreditation in graduate medical education: an antidote to overspecification in the education of medical specialists. *Health Affairs.* 2002; **21**: 103–11.

23 Swanson D, Benbassat J, Bouhuijs P *et al.* Alternative approaches to medical school curricula. In: Page G, ed. *Essays on Curriculum Development and Evaluation in Medicine: report of the Second Cambridge Conference.* Vancouver, BC: Medical School, Coordinator of Health Sciences Office; 1989. pp. 21–34.

24 Boelen C. The five-star doctor. *Acad Med.* 1992; **67**: 745–9.

25 Bligh J, Prideaux D, Parsell G. PRISMS: new educational strategies for medical education. *Med Educ.* 2001; **35**: 520–1.

26 Royal College of Physicians and Surgeons of Canada. *Skills for the New Millennium: report of the societal needs working group. CanMEDS 2000 Project.* Ottawa, ON: Royal College of Physicians and Surgeons of Canada; 2005.

27 Anonymous. *Sheffield Core Curriculum: generic graduate skills.* Sheffield: University of Sheffield; 2003.

28 Anonymous. *Sheffield Core Curriculum.* Sheffield: University of Sheffield; 2003.

29 De Camp K, Vernooij-Dassen MJ, Grol RP *et al.* How to conceptualize professionalism: a qualitative study. *Med Teacher.* 2004; **26**: 696–702.

30 de Cossart L, Fish D. *Cultivating a Thinking Surgeon: new perspectives on clinical teaching, learning and assessment.* Shrewsbury: TFM Publishing; 2005.

31 Leinhardt G, Young KM, Merriman J. Integrating professional knowledge: the theory of practice and the practice of theory. *Learn Instruct.* 1995; **5**: 401–8.

32 Zimmerman BJ. Self-efficacy: an essential motive to learn. *Contemp Educ Psychol.* 2000; **25**: 82–91.

33 Zimmerman BJ. Self-regulation involves more than metacognition: a social cognitive perspective. *Educ Psychol.* 1995; **30**: 217–21.

34 Boekaerts M. Self-regulated learning: where we are today. *Int J Educ Res.* 1999; **31**: 445–57.

35 Miller GE. The assessment of clinical skills/competence/performance. *Acad Med.* 1990; **65**: S63–7.

36 Wenger E. *Communities of Practice: learning, meaning, and identity.* Cambridge: Cambridge University Press; 1998.

37 Campion P, Foulkes J, Neighbour R *et al.* Patient centredness in the MRCGP video examination: analysis of large cohort. *BMJ.* 2002; **325**: 691–2.

38 Irby DM. Teaching and learning in ambulatory care settings: a thematic review of the literature. *Acad Med.* 1995; **70**: 898–931.

39 Parsell G, Bligh J. Recent perspectives on clinical teaching. *Med Educ.* 2001; **35**: 409–14.

40 Jolly B. Historical and theoretical background. In: Jolly B, Rees L, eds. *Medical Education in the Millennium.* Oxford: Oxford University Press; 1998. pp. 171–87.

41 Eraut M, Steadman S. *Early Career Learning in the Professional Workplace: theories, methods and insights from a longitudinal, cross-professional, comparative study.* British Educational Research Association Annual Conference, University of Glamorgan, 2005.

42 Brophy J, Alleman J. Activities as instructional tools: a framework for analysis and evaluation. *Educ Researcher.* 1991; **20:** 9–23.

43 Hafferty F. Beyond curriculum reform: confronting medicine's hidden curriculum. *Acad Med.* 1998; **73:** 403–7.

44 Styles WM. . . . but now what? Some unresolved problems of training for general practice. *Br J Gen Pract.* 1990; **40:** 270.

45 Snyder BR. *The Hidden Curriculum.* New York: Alfred A Knopf; 1970.

46 Haidet P, Stein HF. The role of the student–teacher relationship in the formation of physicians. The hidden curriculum as process. *J Gen Intern Med.* 2006; **21 (Suppl. 1):** S16–20.

47 Hodges B. The many and conflicting histories of medical education in Canada and the USA: an introduction to the paradigm wars. *Med Educ.* 2005; **39:** 613–21.

48 Ozolins I, Hall H, Peterson R. The student voice: recognising the hidden and informal curriculum in medicine. *Med Teacher.* 2008; **30:** 606–11.

49 Singer PA, Wu AW, Fazel S *et al.* An ethical dilemma: Medical errors and medical culture; An error of omission; Commentary: Learning to love mistakes; Commentary: Doctors are obliged to be honest with their patients; Commentary: A climate of secrecy undermines public trust. *BMJ.* 2001; **322:** 1236–40.

50 Hunter KM. *Doctors' Stories: the narrative structure of medical knowledge.* Princeton, NJ: Princeton University Press; 1993.

51 Benner P. From novice to expert. *Am J Nurs.* 1982; **82:** 402–7.

52 Dreyfus HL, Dreyfus SE. Peripheral vision: expertise in real world contexts. *Organization Studies.* 2005; **26:** 779–92.

53 Marinker M. Assessment of postgraduate medical education – future directions. In: Lawrence M, Pritchard P, eds. *General Practitioner Education: UK and Nordic perspectives.* London: Springer Verlag; 1992. pp. 75–80.

54 Young M. Knowledge, learning and the curriculum of the future. *Br Educ Res J.* 1999; **25:** 463–77.

55 Marinker M. The language of medical education. In: Cormack J, Marinker M, Morrell D, eds. *Teaching General Practice.* London: Kluwer Medical; 1981. pp. 7–14.

CHAPTER 8

Matching methods with message

This chapter will help you to choose the teaching method that will most efficiently achieve your learning objectives. The following teaching strategies are considered, with tips for making the best use of them, plus what to consider if they are failing to work:

➤ ad-hoc teaching
➤ teaching a practical skill
➤ giving a lecture
➤ running a workshop
➤ working in small groups
➤ running a learning group
➤ problem-based learning
➤ using audiovisual aids.

The selection and use of educational tools and methods utilising technology are discussed in Chapter 9.

SELECTING TEACHING METHODS

A plethora of teaching methods exist, although not all of them will be relevant for all teachers or situations. As you consider your learners' needs and educational objectives, you will broaden the range of teaching methods and learning strategies that you can offer them. Medical teachers are expected to demonstrate competence in a range of teaching methods and technologies.[1]

In healthcare, all types of learning are possible, including ad-hoc bedside or clinic sessions. All can be planned or prepared for to a greater or lesser extent. Consider the traits of a good teacher, which are listed in Box 8.1.

BOX 8.1 The traits of a good teacher

A good teacher will:
• understand the learner's needs
• set appropriate learning objectives
• prepare well so that the context and content are clear and focused

---

- match educational methods with those objectives
- stimulate the learner
- challenge the learner
- interest the learner
- involve the learner
- encourage the learner – with positive feedback
- use a style of delivery that suits the learner's needs
- evaluate the teaching and the learning
- refine future teaching in the light of the evaluation
- be a lifelong learner.

Ideally, the first step when planning an educational session is to carefully and explicitly define the learning objectives, and then match your teaching strategy with those objectives. For example, if by the end of the course you want learners to be able to swim, you need to teach in a swimming pool. If your objective is to show how much fun swimming is, you could show a video of people in a pool, or you could invite people to share their experiences in a lecture theatre.

Pragmatically, the teaching method is usually dictated, or at least influenced, by the available resources. Often you are invited to give a lecture, so the method is set for you. However, effective teachers show flexibility and creativity. If there is just you, one room and 50 learners you will probably use a lecture format. However, be flexible about the audiovisual equipment that you use and the content and style of handouts. Within a lecture theatre, small group discussions are possible. Ask people to discuss specific points with their neighbour.

AD-HOC TEACHING

Much of your teaching will probably occur while you are working in busy clinical settings. Increasingly, you will come to rely on ad-hoc teaching to cover important issues.

Often learners ask for explanations relating to their experiences as they go along, and you must manage this situation without the luxury of prior research or preparation of visual aids. Prepare for this by having a framework in mind that can be applied as appropriate. The five 'microskills' listed in Box 8.2[2] can help you to assess, instruct and give feedback more efficiently.

BOX 8.2 The one-minute teacher: five microskills for clinical teaching[2]

1 Get a commitment. Ask 'What do you think is going on here?' Ask the learner how they interpreted the situation to establish their learning needs.
2 Probe for supporting evidence. Ask 'What led you to that conclusion?' Ask the learner for their evidence before offering your opinion. This will allow you to find out what they know and identify knowledge gaps.
3 Teach general rules and principles: 'When this happens, do this . . .' Instruction will be better remembered if it is given as a general rule or principle.
4 Reinforce what was right and be specific: 'You did an excellent job of . . .' Learners' skills that are not well established need to be reinforced. Praise motivates people.

5 Correct mistakes: 'Next time this happens, try this instead . . .' Mistakes that are not addressed have a good chance of being repeated.

TEACHING PRACTICAL SKILLS AND TECHNICAL PROCEDURES

All healthcare professionals must learn to perform the various procedures that their daily work involves. This could range from performing a series of specific physical activities in complex and demanding settings (e.g. a neurosurgical operating theatre), through to learning to conduct an effective patient interview, or to perform an efficient, comfortable patient examination or undertake appropriate counselling and psychotherapy sessions.

The environment should provide encouragement and support so that learners can reach the high quality of skills performance that is required to ensure patient safety and optimal health outcomes. The teacher should check that all of the required materials are available and other healthcare professionals can provide necessary support.

Once upon a time, the saying was 'See one, do one, teach one.' Research into improving the performance of athletes, musicians and other trainees now gives us a clearer idea of what works in skills training, and the multiple stages of development required. A seasoned expert is able to create new methods, or at least be able to easily adapt existing procedures, to new or special circumstances.

The cognitive processes of a novice engaging in a practical skill are quite different to those of an expert. The goal of the novice is to achieve competence in the skill and feel comfortably proficient. The expert may think little about each step, but consciously slows down and increases their attentiveness when unexpected challenges arise.

Teachers know that learners must have appropriate knowledge, attitudes and motor skills for a specific procedure. A novice must be able to perceive the various aspects of the procedure before learning to actually do it. You will initially guide learners, allowing them safe opportunities to try the basic steps and to engage in repeated supervised practice.[3] Later, you should provide opportunities to practise the new skill in increasingly complex situations (*see* Box 8.3).

BOX 8.3 The steps of psychomotor skill acquisition
(Simpson's taxonomy)

1 **Perception:** being aware.
2 **Set:** getting ready.
3 **Guided response:** following instructions.
4 **Mechanism:** following habitual steps in action.
5 **Complex response:** demonstrating coordination and efficiency of activity.
6 **Adaptation:** adjusting procedures to new and special circumstances.
7 **Origination:** creating new procedures.

Eventually the learner will develop correct habits from repeated accurate practice, and will be able to mechanically reproduce the expected steps unassisted. With repeated practice the learner will work more quickly in a coordinated time- and energy-efficient manner. By this stage the learner can begin to teach others how to perform this procedure.

Practice involving repetition of errors does not lead to expertise. Therefore even experts at the very top of their career require masterclasses and private coaching.

Several educational models should be considered when teaching a specific practical skill or procedure. One of the most popular models is the *five-step method*[4] (*see* Box 8.4). For short procedures it can be followed directly. Longer, more complicated operations can be broken down into several shorter components and the model then applied for teaching possibly over an entire training programme.

BOX 8.4 Five-step method[3]

Step 1: Overview discussion
The learners' interest is stimulated by discussing why and how the particular procedure fits into healthcare.

Step 2: Demonstration without narration
The teacher shows the procedure completely and accurately at the usual pace of completion without descriptions to watching learners (conversation with the patient and other team members is continued as usual).

Step 3: Demonstration with discussion
The teacher performs the procedure while explaining each action and answering any questions from learners.

Step 4: Demonstration with learner narration
The teacher undertakes the procedure with learners advising the teacher how to perform each action.

Step 5: Learner performs the procedure
The learner performs the procedure with the teacher watching carefully and coaching as necessary.

A similar model from Walker and Peyton has four steps:
1 demonstration by the teacher
2 deconstruction of the task by the teacher into smaller practice components
3 assessing learner comprehension
4 learner performance.

Simulation

Simulation, whether using high-fidelity computerised models or traditional training materials, can be utilised during the early stages of learning before learners practise on real patients. Surgical programmes may require learners to spend the initial months of their training acquiring and demonstrating competence in many of the basic technical skills (e.g. suturing, manipulating endoscopy equipment) in simulation labs before starting to work in the actual operating theatre. This allows repeated practice of diffi-cult technical procedures, thus developing confidence and competence. Patient safety is protected and less time is lost in patient care settings helping novices to learn simple skills. Using simulations allows programme curricula to be designed to incorporate a broad and sequential range of necessary basic skills, and the training tools to be validated and reused.

A similar principle can help learners to transfer skills from one procedure in which they are proficient to another which has related components. For example, dilating the cervix of a patient under anaesthetic prepares a practitioner to insert an intrauterine device into a patient who is awake.

Simulated or standardised patients can be used to help learners to practise history taking, explanation and communication skills. Simulated patients are actors who have rehearsed detailed information in order to accurately portray themselves as patients. Standardised patients are those who truly have a specific condition, and who have been trained to present their condition consistently between learners. Simulated and standardised patients can be trained to provide unique and useful feedback to learners from the patient perspective.

Use of educational technology

Videos can be used to provide demonstrations for steps 2 or 3 of the *five-step method*. These may be available on peer-reviewed educational websites or less officially on universally available websites (e.g. YouTube). Computer gaming software can provide realistic 2-D and 3-D simulations with features such as built-in timers and 'beat-the-clock', to demonstrate increasing speed as competence increases. Learners can review videos of themselves with peers or teachers.

Advance mental practice

Mental practice, or rehearsal in one's mind prior to a performance, can help during both early and later stages of learning. Its effects are primarily in the cognitive and psychological preparedness aspects, rather than in physical muscle reactions.[5]

Use of guidelines

National guidelines can be helpful, and must be followed when learners are practising practical skills. Cutting corners is inappropriate unless a very expert level of practice has been reached.

Assessment of performance

Clinical outcomes can be measured in a number of ways (e.g. through quality assurance systems, clinical audits and other measures of task flow or follow-up).

Benchmarking performance on a scale of skill and against the performance of other professionals, practices or institutions ensures quality assurance and determines whether the skill has been well learned and applied consistently.

GIVING A LECTURE

The advantages of the lecture are well known.
➤ Expertise is shared with many learners within a short period of time.
➤ It is relatively cheap in terms of resources, as one room is used, with one lecturer to many learners.
➤ Quick syllabus coverage can be achieved with a series of lectures.

➤ Expert clarification of difficult concepts can be achieved.
➤ It is a good format for a new topic and/or one about which little has been written.
➤ It allows a more meaningful description of feelings, and the potential for infectious enthusiasm to be transmitted from lecturer to learner, motivating learners to find out more.

However, there are also many disadvantages to the lecture format.
➤ Passivity of the audience may shorten their concentration span to 10 minutes or so.
➤ There is little or no opportunity to ask questions.
➤ Learners' natural reticence prevents them from asking questions, due to fear of appearing stupid.
➤ Information is delivered at the same pace for all learners, which may be too fast or too slow for some audience members.
➤ It is difficult to assess content balance and reliability when faced with a single view of an enthusiastic expert.

Things that can go wrong, so that the delivery of teaching is impaired

- Misjudging learners' prior knowledge – assuming too much or too little.
- Delivery of inappropriate teaching – too fast, boring, monotonous, challenging, funny, or difficult to hear the words clearly.
- Format of teaching is mismatched with learners and/or content, such as a lecture when interaction is required, too little discussion, or small group work that is too threatening.
- Dependence on audiovisual aids, causing panic when they fail to function properly.
- Poor preparation for questions, so that the teacher appears ignorant.
- Lack of familiarity with the venue delaying the presentation while the teacher arranges lighting, seating, ventilation or audiovisual equipment.
- Being late due to not allowing sufficient travelling time.
- Poor lighting – too dark, causing the audience to fall asleep, or too bright, making slides illegible.
- Presentation appears disjointed because it lacks a logical flow.
- Too many speakers are involved, causing confusion to the audience.
- The lecturer looks down, avoids eye contact or continually turns their back to the audience to look at the slides on the screen.
- The topic is so difficult that learners risk leaving the session either ill informed or more confused than they were before.
- Poor time keeping, particularly when the session is part of a tight programme.
- Inadequate structuring around learning outcomes that are relevant, necessary or important to the learners and match their preferences or needs.

You may avoid problems with giving a lecture if you do the following.
➤ Establish the exact nature of the audience and their likely levels of knowledge and experience.

➤ Practise your talk. Time it carefully, making sure that you leave enough time to focus on the main points. Consider recording your practice talk and asking colleagues for constructive comments.

➤ Link your lecture into previous presentations by arriving early enough to hear them or arranging a private briefing from the course organiser before you speak.

➤ Open your lecture by sparking the attention of the audience in some way – with a prop, a challenging remark or a rhetorical question. Do not open by apologising for your lack of knowledge or for being there or keeping them from food, drink or freedom.

➤ 'Say what you are going to say, say it and then repeat what you said', as they say.

➤ Do not anxiously rock backwards and forwards when speaking into a static microphone, or your voice level will ebb and flow.

➤ Arrive early enough to check that your audiovisual aids are functioning and to establish how to operate the controls.

➤ Take a pointer with you in case one is not available at the venue.

➤ Fix your notes together if they are on different cards or pages, to maintain the correct order.

➤ Use a highlighter pen over key points of your lecture notes to enable you to pick out important phrases at a glance.

➤ Regularly raise your eyes to scan around the audience. Fix on one or two people when you are talking. Look at the back rows to prevent them feeling disconnected from the lecture.

➤ Develop your own style. Don't try and be funny if telling jokes makes you quake. Don't be crude or swear in a professional setting.

➤ Wear comfortable and appropriate clothes.

➤ Have water available if you are a nervous speaker.

➤ Write yourself big notices in your lecture notes saying 'slow down' if you tend to speak too fast, or timings if you often run behind schedule.

➤ Place your watch in a prominent position to remind you of the time.

➤ Inform the audience at the start whether you will take questions during or at the end of your lecture.

➤ Think positive, and imagine yourself giving a lecture and everything going well. Exude an air of enthusiasm and confidence about the subject.

➤ Finish with a well-polished, relevant conclusion. Perhaps use the answer to the rhetorical question posed at the beginning, the end of a story that was half told earlier in the presentation, or a challenge or action plan for the future. Don't just tail off and stop abruptly.

Holding your audience

An unresponsive audience can unnerve even experienced teachers. People behave differently when speaking in a one-to-one situation from when they give a lecture to a large number of people or run a workshop with groups of more than four or six people.[4] In normal conversation the listener actively supports and encourages the speaker by giving non-verbal signs, making a suggestion if the speaker is lost for a word, and synchronising facial expressions and body posture with what the speaker is saying. When a lecturer addresses a large audience this supportive interaction is lost and audience behaviour may even be offputting. Learners' stares can seem threatening rather than the expressions of concentration which they might be. You may mistakenly interpret uninhibited comfort movements (e.g. head-propping, shuffling and yawning) as signs of boredom and disrespect. Neill termed this 'diffusion of responsibility' with 'no one responsible for supporting and providing feedback to the speaker, who may feel, from the lack of apparent response, as if he or she is throwing stones into treacle.'[6]

After a few minutes audiences tend to relax and display inattentive behaviour. When audiences are primed to put lecturers off by appearing to be inattentive, lecturers tend to perform worse than when audiences are primed to appear supportive and interested. To some extent, audiences should take responsibility for the quality of the lecture that they receive. Expect this type of behaviour, and either resolve not to be put off by it or take it personally and press on regardless despite the lack of feedback or support, or actively engage the audience by asking them questions, triggering discussion, setting challenges and using other interactive exercises.

RUNNING A WORKSHOP

A workshop format is useful if you want to exchange ideas and experiences about a relatively new area. It encourages interaction and discussion in response to a short, targeted expert input. A workshop relies on learners being willing to contribute and to think about how what they have heard applies to their situation and justify why they may or may not make changes. Workshops sometimes follow a didactic lecture, providing the audience with an opportunity to think the topic through and challenge the speaker. If a workshop stands alone, the workshop leader will usually give a short presentation to introduce the subject and discussion points. Sometimes a workshop format is used for classroom teaching, such as learning critical appraisal skills or learning how to use new computer software. In these cases the leader often remains as an instructor and responds to questions throughout the session.

You may avoid problems with running a workshop by doing the following.

➤ Choose a title that is explicit and unambiguous, so that learners are unlikely to be misled about its content.

➤ Ensure that learners receive an abstract of the workshop prior to the session and are well primed about the topic and content of the workshop and the backgrounds of the facilitator(s).

➤ Hold a practice session first, especially if there is more than one workshop facilitator, to make sure that the facilitators share the same approach to the workshop, understand the learning objectives, agree roles and responsibilities, have small group facilitation skills and keep to time.

➤ Plan and keep to a timetable. Place it in a prominent position so that you and the other speakers or facilitators can keep an eye on the time. Be in a position to alert speakers who run over time.

➤ Establish the nature and likely prior knowledge of the audience.

➤ Inform the course or conference organiser of the upper limit of numbers of learners for your workshop prior to the event.

➤ Produce a sufficient number of copies of the small group discussion topics, so that delegates can remind themselves easily about the nature of the task in hand.

➤ Arrange for a flipchart with plenty of paper to be available for each small group. Take spare flipchart pens. Take Blu-Tack® to help you to display flipchart reports to all learners.
➤ If the workshop involves representatives of small groups feeding back what they have discussed, make sure that these reporters keep to time and stay focused on presenting the discussion of their tasks.
➤ Round up the final plenary discussion with a conclusion based on the small group discussions that relates back to the objective of the workshop.

Things that can go wrong with small group functioning

- Groups are not well balanced (e.g. everyone sticks with friends or close colleagues instead of mixing with others). This can stifle discussion and limit the exchange of ideas.
- Members of the group do not introduce themselves, so no one knows who anyone is or what their backgrounds are.
- Conduct rules about confidentiality or the boundaries of discussion are not discussed or agreed, so that people feel they cannot speak about sensitive information. Even worse, group members confide sensitive information which is subsequently relayed outside the group.
- Too many small groups are packed into one room, so group members have difficulty hearing what others are saying and are distracted by what other groups are doing.
- Too little time is allowed for the small group discussion, preventing all of the tasks from being addressed.
- One or two members dominate the group while others sit quietly and unengaged.
- At the report-back session the group member presents their own views instead of the essence of the group's discussions.

SMALL GROUP TEACHING
Why use small group teaching?

Small groups encourage learners to interact, explore and develop ideas. You might run a small group after a lecture, to allow the learners to debate the points that they have just heard, the extent to which these apply to their own circumstances and how they could change their professional practice or personal behaviour in response. A small group might be a forum for the exchange of different ideas to help learners to share tips and experiences that stimulate reflection and forward thinking. Small group work encourages learners to think independently, develop their own ideas and challenge preconceived beliefs. This is active learning, and it is often more effective than more passive methods (e.g. lectures).

Small group work promotes critical and logical thinking as part of a problem-solving approach. You might also consider using small group work to build up a team to help group members to understand why other members hold different views and what makes them tick.

Small group work is usually based on a task that is wide enough to encourage the learners to own and develop the topic themselves, but focused enough to restrict the ensuing discussions to the matter in hand. In small group work it is the learners who are key to the subsequent discussion, rather than the facilitator, whose opinions are of lesser or no importance.

If there is sufficient time, a small group evolves through five stages of development in group dynamics.[7]

1 **Forming:** getting to know one another.
2 **Norming:** the norms, roles and goals of the group are worked out through informal discussion, possibly checking out the task with the facilitator. There may be expressions of uncertainty about the task and some frustrations about lack of progress.
3 **Storming:** leaders emerge and some learners are perceived by the other group members as having special talents. There may be emotion, anger and impatience, requiring facilitation skills to hold the group together.
4 **Performing:** decisions are reached, and tasks are sorted out with a lot of mutual support and individual satisfaction. The group ends by reviewing and summarising its achievements.
5 **Mourning:** the group begins to disband as time runs out and members reluctantly leave the group. The facilitator may need to lighten the gloom and bereavement responses at this stage.

You may avoid problems with small group teaching by doing the following.
➤ Limit the numbers in a small group to 12, but preferably six or eight.
➤ Arrange the chairs facing each other in a circle, so that all members feel equally part of the group and can easily see everyone else.
➤ Remove any empty chairs so that the group feels complete.
➤ Appoint a facilitator who is skilled at handling group dynamics.
➤ Start the small group work by welcoming everybody, to create a positive atmosphere. Introduce yourself and ask the others to do the same.
➤ Agree ground rules about confidentiality at the beginning, and listen respectfully to each others' views and comments.
➤ Ensure that everyone knows what the task(s) involve. Have plenty of copies of the task(s) written out, or display them on a flipchart or project them from a computer.
➤ Brief the facilitator so that they know what main points should emerge and can guide the group members back to the central task if they become side-tracked.
➤ Encourage a group member to report the group's discussion back at a subsequent plenary session. Choose this person at the beginning so that they have ample warning and can take notes of everyone's contribution. This discourages reliance on the facilitator and maximises the engagement of the learners in addressing the task.
➤ If asked for information or an opinion, the facilitator should reflect questions back to the group rather than being seen to act as an expert.
➤ Ensure that everyone has a chance to have a say and contribute (*see* Chapter 17 for tips).
➤ Keep to time. The facilitator should have a general sense of the time allocated for each stage of the expected discussion, and should move the group on accordingly so that there is sufficient time to talk about alternative solutions and reach conclusions. Leave five minutes at the end so that the reporter can write down the main points for presenting at the plenary session.

Things that can go wrong with a learning group

- All of the problems and issues listed in the section on 'small group' work.
- Members do not prioritise group meetings, and send last-minute apologies for their absence.
- The facilitator is not skilled enough to 'control' bombastic members who inappropriately dominate the quieter ones.
- The group appears purposeless, without a defined curriculum.
- Alternatively, the opposite may occur, with the prescriptive curriculum stifling exploratory discussions and development.
- Members have false expectations of what being in the group means, and want more direction, networking or support than is on offer.
- Insufficient effort is put into the 'forming' stage of the group to build sound relationships, respect and mutual understanding.
- The facilitator interferes too much in the group's development, and it is unclear whether they are a group member or not.
- There is too much external input and insufficient time to make the most of group members' potential contributions.
- Personalities clash and members don't gel, creating friction and frustration within the group, which boil over and disrupt progress in discussions.

RUNNING A LEARNING GROUP

There is confusion about the terms 'learner set', 'learning group', 'learner group' and 'action learner set', and no general consensus about the different meanings of these names or types of group.

A 'learning group' format is a variety of 'small group' where the members meet regularly over time. It usually refers to a group of people who meet with the common aim of enhancing their personal and/or professional development by learning from each other. If the main purpose is to improve personal development, this might include learning more from each other about boosting self-confidence, self-esteem and personal presentation skills, as well as increasing achievement and career progression. If professional development is the main purpose, the group might be more topic-based around healthcare service management or organisational issues. Groups that are established for peer support (e.g. Balint groups, where members discuss particular doctor–patient relationship issues on an ongoing basis) are another type of 'learning group', but are not discussed further here.

A learning group facilitator has to be especially skilled in group dynamics, as learning groups often consist of those who have already achieved a great deal in their own field and want to develop themselves and their ideas further. Such people may be used to authoritative roles in their workplaces and struggle to leave this position behind, listen attentively to others and consider peers as equals. Because of the members' backgrounds, little external input should be necessary, as members should be willing to impart their considerable previous experience, knowledge and skills to others.

A learning group should enable participants to develop their own learning needs with regard to their own individual needs and the organisation's needs. It should assist members through varied learning support mechanisms to meet their learning needs. Within a healthcare service, learning groups consisting of a mix of healthcare professionals can be set up to enhance understanding of each others' roles and responsibilities, and to promote respect for the skills and strengths of colleagues from other disciplines.

You may avoid problems with learning groups by doing the following.

➤ Issue a learning group charter or contract with the invitation to potential members to join, explaining the purpose and nature of the learning group format.

➤ Only invite people to join the learning group if they are likely to get on with other members and are at similar stages of their personal and/or professional development.

➤ Make the establishment of good relationships within the group a priority at the first meeting. This may involve agreeing and owning group rules, encouraging group members to regard each other as peers whatever their professional status or position, and taking time for members to introduce themselves as individuals.

➤ Clarify the role of the facilitator in relation to being a group member, providing expertise, and arranging hospitality and meetings.

➤ Fix dates for meetings well in advance, so that members have the maximum opportunity to attend.

➤ Hold learning group meetings when the members are most likely to attend and feel relaxed. For example, full-day meetings avoid work being squeezed in around them, or late-afternoon meetings can end with a meal to encourage further networking between members.

➤ Accept that learning group members can gain technical knowledge elsewhere and that the two main purposes of the group are to learn more about the 'softer' aspects of personal and professional development, such as attitudes, feelings, relationships and values, and to give each other peer support.

➤ Agree some outcomes of the learning group so that members can gauge whether they are making progress and whether their time is being wisely invested.

PROBLEM-BASED LEARNING

Problem-based learning (PBL) is a form of group working that can powerfully facilitate active learning. It requires attention to particular aspects of learner study skills, a high degree of learner self-directedness, excellent facilitation skills and an understanding of the process by the teachers.

PBL reverses the traditional approach to teaching and learning. It starts with individual examples or problems, through the consideration of which learners develop general principles and concepts that they can generalise to other situations (*see* Table 8.1).[8]

PBL can result in:

➤ deep learning

➤ learners activating prior learning and integrating new knowledge with it

➤ lifelong learning skills

➤ generic competences (e.g. collaboration)

➤ learners assisting each other to find ways to understand and retain knowledge

➤ the sharing of useful sources of information.

TABLE 8.1 Steps in the problem-based learning process as applied to a specific example

The group clarifies the text of the problem scenario	The mother of a 13-year-old girl phones the surgery to ask the receptionist whether her daughter has been seen that day by a doctor
Learners define the problem	Isn't that confidential information?
Brainstorming is used to identify possible explanations/solutions	The girl is under-age, so the mother must be worried
	The girl might never come to the doctor again if she thinks we tell her mother everything
	Should that be something the receptionist deals with or the doctor?
Group reaches interim conclusion	It is an ethical/medico-legal dilemma
Group formulates learning objectives	To find out what the law says
	To find out what ethicists think
	To find out what doctors say in real life
Learners go away and work independently to achieve the learning outcomes	Library visits, Internet searches, interviews with practitioners, discussion among peers, friends and family
Group reconvenes to discuss the knowledge acquired	Pooling of results and sources. Tutor checks learning, clarifies and corrects if necessary

How to create effective PBL scenarios
➤ Learning objectives must be defined in advance.
➤ Problems should be appropriate to the stage of the curriculum and the learners' level of understanding.
➤ Scenarios should be relevant to practice.
➤ Problems should be presented in context to encourage integration of knowledge.
➤ Scenarios should present cues to stimulate discussion and encourage learners to seek an explanation.
➤ Each problem should be of sufficient depth to prevent too early resolution.
➤ Learners should be actively engaged in searching for information.

Disadvantages of PBL[9]
➤ Learners may feel 'all at sea' if the process is not managed and introduced well and/or they are unprepared for such self-directedness.
➤ Facilitators may not have the competences to manage PBL, particularly if they were taught according to a traditional curriculum.
➤ Facilitators may resent not being able to 'teach' (i.e. transfer their knowledge and understanding).
➤ The knowledge gained can be disorganised, and important information may not be identified as such. Good tutoring is required to address this during the group discussion of knowledge acquired.

➤ Learners may fail to identify all of the necessary points from the case, and thus fail to learn parts of the curriculum.
➤ More staff and resources may be needed to support and facilitate the sessions and the resulting searches.
➤ Learners may miss out on role modelling from inspirational teachers.

Many of these disadvantages can be addressed through training and preparation of both learners and tutors.

EQUIPMENT AND VISUAL AIDS

Teachers should use any audiovisual aids that will enhance the delivery of their material, reinforce their messages and command the learners' attention. However, if you are totally reliant on audiovisual equipment, consider what you will do if it fails to work.

Using a flipchart

A flipchart allows small groups to identify and record their concerns and ideas as they arise. As the pages are filled, they can be posted around the room so that the learners can refer to earlier suggestions and ideas. The flipchart is a useful interactive educational tool so long as the scribe faces the other learners and doesn't just list their own ideas.

If you plan to write a lot as a teacher, a flipchart may be the wrong tool. You may wish to write on acetates on an overhead projector so that you can develop your argument while facing the group.

Always carry a flipchart pen. You never know when you might want to capture the content of discussions on a flipchart or whiteboard (for the latter, make sure that your pen has water-soluble ink).

PowerPoint presentations

Information on the uses and drawbacks of PowerPoint presentations can be found in Chapter 9. Tips for 'effective PowerPoint presentations for the technologically challenged'[10] include practical advice on storyboarding, the size of fonts, the use of colour and common pitfalls. Also consider the following.
➤ Prepare a structured framework for the content. Create a 'storyboard' that takes you logically through the content, from objectives through the main content material, concluding with learning points.
➤ Choose a format that is appropriate to the theme of your talk. Be alert to the right ratio of illustrative graphs, complementary clip art, and sound and video linked to your presentation as appropriate. Only include such extras if they enhance the educational delivery.
➤ Use clear, legible text in short phrases or sentences to aid the viewers' understanding and keep their attention.
➤ Employ a sans-serif font such as Arial, where the letters have no tail, as these are less decorative and therefore more easily read on the screen.
➤ Match the font size to the size of the lecture room, from a 36 point size text in lecture theatres with more than 200 seats down to a 24 point size in classrooms with less than 50 seats.
➤ Include a maximum of one idea or point per screen.

➤ Limit yourself to six or fewer words per line in six or fewer lines.
➤ Use predominantly lower-case letters, as they are more comprehensible to the reader. Restrict capitals to headings.
➤ Do not overuse colour. Stick to a maximum of four colours on any one screen, and be consistent with what different colours represent throughout your presentation.
➤ Make sure that your text is legible against your background. Maximise the contrast between text and background colours.
➤ Check that colours look the same when projected on to a screen.
➤ Check that your computer output is compatible with the equipment and software at the venue.
➤ Always have a back-up in case technology fails you.
➤ Rehearse the presentation to ensure that you keep to time without moving through the slides too quickly. Ensure that you are giving learners enough opportunity to read and digest your slides as well as hear what you are saying
➤ Know and plan how you will operate the computer.
➤ Prepare complementary handouts. Find the *handout* print option that enables you to print the slides on the left-hand side of the sheet of paper, leaving room for notes and questions on the right-hand side.
➤ Place a logo in the same position on each slide to give the impression of a coherent presentation.

Overhead slides

Although PowerPoint is increasingly the visual method of choice, overhead projectors are still found in some educational settings. For pre-prepared overhead slides you should follow the points covered above about text size, design, colour and format. Unless you are using overhead slides to write down the group's ideas as they produce them, prepare your overhead slides well so that they are attractive, neat and command the attention of your audience.

Consider using plastic pockets to file and protect your overheads. Take acetates out of the pocket when showing them at the presentation, to prevent blurring.

Be careful to use the correct type of heat-resistant overhead film if you are using an inkjet printer or photocopier machine. The wrong type of film may melt inside a printer/photocopier and stop it from functioning.

Tips from experienced teachers

When considering which teaching method to use, try asking yourself the following questions.

- What are the learners' objectives?
- What am I trying to achieve? What are my objectives?
- Is this the best way of achieving them?
- What other ways are there of achieving them?
- What are the strengths of the way I have chosen?
- What are the potential weaknesses that I will have to be on guard for as facilitator?
- How will I know that this way is the most appropriate way – for me and my learners?
- How will I assess whether the objectives have been achieved?

Audiovisual presentations

Video clips distract the audience. For example, if the equipment fails to work or causes a delay it can disrupt the flow of your presentation. If you do show a video, explain the points of interest before you show it, and then expand on what the viewers will have noticed after they have finished watching it. Use short clips to maintain the momentum of the presentation. You can either use a separate video or DVD player or, to minimise the risk of equipment failure, incorporate the clip into your PowerPoint presentation. If you are linking a clip from a separate file into the presentation, make sure that this works away from the computer on which you created the presentation, as such links sometimes become corrupt.

If you are giving a lecture overseas, make sure that your equipment will be compatible with the audiovisual systems that are provided.

Any patient who appears on an educational video must give informed consent to be filmed and know the context in which you will be using and showing the video.

Information on podcasts can be found in Chapter 9.

REFERENCES

1 Academy of Medical Educators. *Professional Standards*. London: Academy of Medical Educators; 2009.
2 Gordon K, Meyer B, Irby D. *The One Minute Preceptor: five microskills for clinical teaching.* Seattle: University of Washington; 1996.
3 Grantcharov TP, Reznick RK. Teaching procedural skills. *BMJ.* 2008; **336**: 1129–31.
4 George JH, Doto FX. A simple five-step method for teaching clinical skills. *Fam Med.* 2001; **33**: 577–8.
5 Feltz DL, Landers DM. The effects of mental practice on motor skill learning and performance: a meta-analysis. *J Sport Psychol.* 1983; **5**: 25–57.
6 Neill S. In the stare of ravens. *Times Higher Educ.* 1999: **11 June:** 33.
7 Crosby J. *AMEE Medical Education Guide No. 8. Learning in Small Groups.* Dundee: Centre for Medical Education, University of Dundee; 1997.
8 Davis MH, Harden RM. *AMEE Medical Education Guide No. 15. Problem-Based Learning: a practical guide.* Dundee: Centre for Medical Education, University of Dundee; 1999.
9 Wood D. ABC of learning and teaching in medicine: problem-based learning. *BMJ.* 2003; **326**: 328–30.
10 Holzl J. Twelve tips for effective PowerPoint presentations for the technologically challenged. *Med Teacher.* 1997; **19**: 175–9.

FURTHER READING

• Centre for Excellence in Enquiry-Based Learning. www.campus.manchester.ac.uk/ceebl
• Learning Through Enquiry Alliance. www.ltea.ac.uk
• Maskell P. *Working in Groups: a quick guide.* Cambridge: Daniels; 1995.

CHAPTER 9

E-learning and virtual learning environments

Stephen Bostock

E-learning is learning using any type of computer-based technology, but it often refers to the use of online resources or tools accessed through the World Wide Web. This includes access to general information sources (e.g. Wikipedia), academic and special-ist learning resources (e.g. Internet for Midwifery), multimedia such as audio podcasts, as well as tools such as online discussion boards, wikis for collaborative writing, and so on. Business 'productivity' tools, email, presentation software and word processing are also widely used in education. This chapter describes some common uses of these learning technologies and some issues relating to their use.

In the UK, the term *virtual learning environment (VLE)* refers to an integrated collection of online tools for teachers and learners to perform many of the common educational activities traditionally undertaken face to face and on paper.[1] Common examples are Moodle and Blackboard. Their advantages are that, being under institutional control, they are stable, supported and covered by institutional data protection policies. They integrate, into a single site with a consistent interface, many commonly needed course elements such as resource files, web links, on-screen assessments and discussion boards (described below). A disadvantage is that they can never include the most recent tech-nical features available on the public Web. Nonetheless, if you have one, use it!

It used to be assumed that learning online would be a feature of distance learning courses (replacing paper), but in fact technology is more widely used alongside tradi-tional learning and teaching, face to face and paper based, to create 'blended learning.'[2] The degree of online and face-to-face activity in a course varies, but the two modes need to complement and reinforce each other.

Technology has often been called a Trojan horse for pedagogy. When only tradi-tional teaching methods were used, both learners and teachers assumed that they knew, for example, what a lecture was for. Now online alternatives to lectures are available (e.g. digital slides, video, audio, audio over slides). When selecting a technology, you need to question its advantages and disadvantages for your specific context (subject, learners, programme, etc.), and what traditional methods the technology may replace. Using technology thus requires a more thoughtful and systematic selection and design of teaching methods, both technology based and traditional, if they are to be individu-ally effective for learning and mutually reinforcing.

Young adult learners are 'digital natives' – they cannot remember a world before networked computing, they probably own a laptop *and* a smart phone, and they routinely use email, text messaging, online chat, and social networking websites. Although familiar with technology, learners will require you to explain its purpose in their course.

Rather than organising examples of learning technologies by their technical characteristics, this chapter considers common educational activities and suggests how some technologies can be useful. This is inevitably messy, because some educational activities can use a wide range of technologies and, conversely, some technologies are useful for a range of activities.[3] Furthermore, new technologies and new uses for them continually arise, so specific examples soon become out of date! However, the principles of selecting technologies and designing their use will continue to apply.

PRESENTING INFORMATION

Teachers often give presentations of information, and it is common to show slides (e.g. with PowerPoint) from a computer with a digital projector (also *see* Chapter 8). This provides a structure to what you say and allows you to show quotations, pictures, audio or video. One risk of slides is that too much content is shown, too quickly. Learners are trying to listen, watch the screen and (hopefully) make notes. Merely placing content on the screen does little to help learners understand it. Furthermore, slides full of content can become the teacher's autocue – guaranteed to bore! Avoid using built-in graphical features such as patterned backgrounds and animated text, as they often distract and hinder learning.

Digital slides or handouts can easily be made available to learners on a course website or VLE. Consider making them available in advance so that learners can prepare and bring a handout to class if you are not providing one, unless this would spoil a planned surprise element. In the latter case, provide them immediately afterwards. Providing lecture slides and course notes electronically has been disparagingly termed 'shovelware', but learners find it valuable, and often expect it.

As an alternative to PowerPoint you could show web pages or Word documents on the screen, but make sure that the text is large enough (generally 24 point). Another display option is http://prezi.com, which allows you to organise your content as a visual cluster and then zoom into the detail as you want it.

PROVIDING RESOURCES FOR INDIVIDUAL STUDY

The Web can be used to give learners further resources for learning, as pictures, audio or video. However, 'resource-based learning' needs learners to perform purposeful activities with this content, so set clear learning tasks and provide a support system in case of problems. To minimise technical problems, provide the content in common file formats (*see* Box 9.1), and check that all your learners have been able to access it.

Creating multimedia content is now easy. Audio files are often called 'podcasts' (although technically this also involves using a web feed like 'really simple syndication'[4]). They can be recorded on simple digital recorders or on a computer with a microphone. Minimise background noise from the computer and the environment. Recordings of up to five minutes are good for introducing a lecture or providing feedback on questions or coursework. Recordings of whole lectures can be useful for learners to replay while watching your slides online. Creating video is a little more complex, but 'Flip' video cameras are cheap and easy to use. Many digital cameras will capture video. Although the production quality does not need to be top standard, mounting the camera on a simple tripod vastly improves the recording.

BOX 9.1 Common and useful file formats

For text, .rtf is read by all word processors and .htm is read by all browsers. Acrobat .pdf files are also common, but learners must download and install the free Acrobat Reader software (http://get.adobe.com/reader/).

For images, .png is the best general-purpose format, but .jpg is also readable by web browsers, and it is the format created by most digital cameras.

For audio and video, the choice of file format is more complex and there is more risk of problems. Mp3 is widely used for audio and mp4 for video. Flash is widely used for video on the Web, but learners must download and install the free Flash Player (http://get. adobe.com/flashplayer/).

If you use ready-made content, be aware of copyright restrictions.[5] You can provide access to many existing digital resources by providing links to them (URLs), embedded in your website or VLE. Alternatively, you can maintain a list of links to useful web resources on a social bookmarking service such as delicious.com,[6] and reuse it in several courses. A good place to start looking for quality-assured content without copyright problems is Intute.[7] You can also provide your reading lists as web pages with links to texts, electronic journal articles, ebooks (if your institution has them) or digitised content (many universities have a licence from the Copyright Licensing Agency to digitise some existing paper content for courses). Your institution may have centralised reading list software to help you to create electronic reading lists that may improve usage.

Although most learners now use a word processor, this creates only a local file. A blog is a web page that a learner can write, often as a diary or journal, without any technical expertise, and which can then be read by other learners or teachers. An e-portfolio (e.g. Pebblepad) extends this idea to provide an online space where a learner can create a website of web pages, blogs and linked files, and give access to it for particular individuals, such as their tutor or potential employer. Institutional VLEs and e-portfolios often provide blogs, and there are many free blogging services (e.g. www.blogger.com). If you want learners to create learning journals or portfolios, you should consider blogs and e-portfolios.

USING MODELS AND SIMULATIONS

Simulations and models are a category of software that can provide powerful learning environments. A simple numerical example is the use of an MSExcel worksheet to model the growth of a human population. A model has one or more inputs, such as age of first reproduction and infant mortality rate, and one or more outputs, such as population size and age profile. Equations in the worksheet connect the inputs to the outputs. Learners can first enter different values for the inputs (perhaps using data for different developing countries) to observe the predicted population sizes and demography.

Models are simplified versions of reality. Learners can be asked to compare the model's predictions with actual historical data and improve the model, perhaps by adding additional factors using more inputs or modifying the equations. This is a powerful way of understanding population growth. Creating such a spreadsheet model is not difficult once the learner is familiar with spreadsheet software.

A virtual reality simulation relies on realistic audio and video to help learners to imagine and respond to relevant aspects of their environment. For example, a 'virtual patient' on the screen can be programmed to have symptoms of a wide range of ailments for diagnosis.[8] Although this is less realistic than a real patient, or a human actor, it can provide many varied experiences to many learners, to allow them to practise diagnosis repeatedly and when they need to – the software simulation is 'scalable' as a learning environment. If you have the use of an appropriate simulation, it is well worth considering. However, simulations are very costly to produce, and require detailed knowledge of the subject and considerable technical skills, so they are well beyond the scope of individual teachers.

HELPING LEARNERS TO COLLABORATE

Modern theories of learning emphasise both individual intellectual activity and the social context of learning. Learners learn from each other informally, but you can structure collaboration for specific learning purposes. Although learners may be able to meet face to face, there are advantages of textual 'discussions' online, on a private 'discussion board.' This is available any time, anywhere, over an extended period. Messages remain for the period of the course, for group members to read and re-read. There is no limit on 'space', and files can be attached to messages. The software provides tools to help individuals to organise messages as they choose, or to find particular messages. Teachers can control the group composition and monitor individuals' activity in relation to contribution to the discussion. Online textual 'discussion' proceeds much more slowly than verbal discussion, typically over weeks, so their structure must be planned in advance.[9] However, this slower pace means that learners have time to think before contributing. In face-to-face discussions some learners may be unwilling or unable to take a turn in contributing to the continuous flow. Some disadvantages of online collaboration are listed in Box 9.2.

BOX 9.2 Disadvantages of online collaboration

- Some learners may not have easy access to the web server supporting the discussion (e.g. from home).
- Learners may forget their login details.
- Initial unfamiliarity with the system features may slow down or demotivate learners' participation.
- Some learners may be reluctant to contribute such permanent messages, yet read what others write ('lurking'). This may or may not be acceptable, depending on the set task.
- Learners are unlikely to engage unless participation is clearly helpful to passing the course. Make the purpose of discussion clear, or directly assessed.

Just as face-to face discussions or debates can be used as role plays of professional activities, so online textual discussions can be used to simulate some situations for which the course is preparing learners, especially as many professional activities now take place through email messages.

Learner online collaboration can go further than discussion boards. Many systems allow file sharing and shared editing. Whereas a blog is written by one person and made available to others, a wiki allows groups of people to collectively edit one or more documents and link them together. This can be used to support group projects – for example, leading to a collectively written report. The wiki[10] tracks each user's contribution, so the teacher has an audit trail of the group process.

INTERACTING WITH LARGE GROUPS

One view is that teaching is essentially a personal dialogue with learners, and technology can support that dialogue[11] using the tools already mentioned, such as email, discussion boards and blogs. Within a VLE, teachers can make 'announcements' that go to all learners, as institutions will provide class emailing lists. When learners use email or other text communications with teachers, they may not realise the change in tone that is appropriate in an academic context compared with writing to family or friends. Tell them what you expect; effective communication skills require an understanding of the audience. When you write to learners, use a clear, friendly but formal tone. This is professional, not social, and learners need to appreciate this issue for employment. Similarly, online text discussions with other learners as part of coursework should observe 'netiquette' so as not to offend or confuse others.[12]

As the size of the learner group increases, interacting with each individual becomes more difficult in the classroom. Electronic voting handsets, or 'clickers', are a popular and effective means of creating interaction with the whole group.[13] A computer with a projector display must have a radio receiver and appropriate software installed so that, when each learner presses a button on their handset, the computer detects their choice and displays the aggregated votes as a bar chart or pie chart. With most systems (e.g. TurningPoint), the questions must be multiple choice. A simple strategy is to test understanding every 10 or 15 minutes throughout a lecture. If most of the learners fail, there is no point proceeding until the problem has been addressed! More interesting uses can include voting for conflicting views on a contentious issue, which can be discussed in small groups once the learners have decided and communicated their initial view.[14]

The practical disadvantage of clickers, apart from their considerable cost, is that the computer must be ready and the handsets must be distributed and collected. Information 'coverage' is reduced, but this is not a disadvantage if the learners did not previously understand the information given. For large groups the benefits in terms of learner engagement and learner–teacher feedback far outweigh the cost in time. If the technology is not available, a low-technology alternative is the card 'communicubes', which require no technical support, never fail, and are much cheaper.[15]

ASSESSING AND GIVING FEEDBACK

Assessment is a special kind of interaction with learners. It can be summative, giving a grade, or formative, giving feedback on the learner's performance, or both (*see*

Chapter 14). Many courses now assess (grade) learners using coursework. The traditional process was for the learner to word process, print and submit a paper copy, which the teacher would then grade, write feedback on, and return. There are now various technology-based, and hybrid, alternatives. A learner can submit the word-processed file to an electronic 'drop box' from where a marker collects it, annotates it electronically with feedback, and returns it to the drop box for electronic collection. Simultaneously, the teacher provides a grade to an electronic grade book that the learner may access in due course. Anonymity and second marking are possible. A hybrid process involves submission of both an electronic copy and a paper copy. The paper copy is marked and returned with feedback, while the electronic copy is archived, but is available in cases of suspected plagiarism.

The frequency of plagiarism in coursework has increased during the last 20 years, partly because technology makes it easier. The best defence against plagiarism is the better design of assignments,[16] but another tool is text-matching software (e.g. Turnitin[17]). Learners submit their files and teachers mark them, as described above, but they are simultaneously checked for matching text on the Web, in electronic journals, in electronic copies of textbooks, and in the software's database of all learner work submitted to it. Routine submission of coursework to text-matching software is a disincentive to the tiny minority of learners who might cheat. It can also be used educationally, by allowing learners to see the 'originality report' for a draft of their own work. This makes clearer, in a personal, 'concrete' example, the ideas of plagiarism and the proper acknowledgement of sources – crucial topics when educating learners about academic writing.

Computer-based assessment traditionally meant multiple-choice quizzes, or other forms of 'objective tests', conducted on the computer screen. There are many systems available, and all VLEs include one. The computer does the grading, but this is not free – the teacher's effort has been transferred from doing the grading to creating the tests, so the computer can later do the grading automatically. Writing valid, reliable, objective tests is difficult. Their use for summative assessment should be limited to testing introductory, factual material in large classes (where the initial development time can be justified). However, a better use of on-screen tests is to provide formative feedback to learners, on demand. Many learners find such tests helpful and motivating,[18] and tests for this purpose are easier to write – if the validity or reliability is not perfect that is no great problem, if the purpose is to provide feedback.

Providing timely, informative feedback is increasingly highlighted as a part of teaching that is lacking. Feedback may be narrowly regarded, by teachers and learners, as the written comments on a returned piece of coursework, but in fact it is much broader than this (*see* Chapter 13). Learning requires information on current performance and guidance on how to improve it. Providing more traditional face-to-face or written feedback is not scalable for large classes, but technology can help. For example, feedback as a numbered list of common deficiencies, and suggestions for their improvement, can be emailed to the whole class, with specific numbered points sent to each individual. Electronic submissions can be marked by annotating the learner's file (e.g. in Word using 'insert comment' or 'track changes') or in Turnitin's online marking tool, Grademark. This can reduce turn-around times and streamline the process. It also avoids the common complaint of illegible handwritten comments.

A more recent innovation is the use of digital audio feedback. Using the technology described above, this can provide more information (in voice tone), and takes no longer to create than written feedback. In large cohorts it may be a good alternative to providing individual feedback tutorials. If it *is* possible to offer a short face-to-face meeting to provide feedback, making an audio recording of the meeting (or allowing the learner to do this) provides a record to which the learner can return for confirmation and further understanding.

One technology that has not yet been mentioned is screencasting. Using either PC software (e.g. Camtasia) or free web services (e.g. jing.com or screenr.com), the moving computer screen is captured along with a verbal commentary of up to five minutes. The screen can show the learner coursework, with highlights added to focus the attention on aspects being discussed in the verbal feedback. With a little practice, this takes no longer than writing the feedback, and provides more information and personal contact.

WHICH SOFTWARE?

Some learning technologies are part of a VLE, which provides them in a stable, supported, integrated environment within an institution. Other technologies may not be available within your institution, but may be available as free services on the Web. Whether you should use these free services depends on a number of factors. For example, European data protection laws mean that any personal data, including learner names, should not be placed in most IT systems outside Europe. Furthermore, systems in the USA are subject to the Patriot Act, and may be open to the security services. Free web services may disappear without notice, or require you to pay. Therefore for 'high-risk', graded work you should only use institutional systems or ask for advice. However, for optional, informal group discussions or support, a social networking (e.g. Facebook) group may be familiar and preferable to learners who would not use the discussion board in your VLE unless it was a course requirement.

MOBILE LEARNING

The continuing development of mobile, networked devices is creating increasing possibilities for 'mobile learning'. The range of devices already includes laptop/notebook PCs, netbooks, handheld PCs, mobile phones, iPhones and other smart phones, iPods, e-readers and iPads. As Wi-Fi hotspots proliferate and phone networks improve, these devices will be permanently 'connected'. New opportunities will arise for designing and supporting active and social learning, and we shall need to be creative in grasping them.

REFERENCES

1 Bostock SJ. VLEs – don't panic. *Educ Developments*. 2003; 4.4: 28. www.seda.ac.uk/index. php?p=5_4_1
2 MacDonald J. *Blended Learning and Online Tutoring*. 2nd edn. Aldershot: Gower; 2008.
3 Bostock SJ. *e-Teaching: engaging learners through technology*. London: Staff and Educational Development Association; 2007.
4 http://en.wikipedia.org/wiki/RSS
5 www.keele.ac.uk/library/support/copyright/
6 http://delicious.com/stephen_bostock/blended_learning

7 www.intute.ac.uk

8 www.keele.ac.uk/pharmacy/vp/

9 Salmon G. *E-tivities*. London: RoutledgeFalmer; 2002. Support website is available at www. atimod.com/e-tivities/intro.shtml

10 http://PBworks.com

11 Laurillard D. *Rethinking University Teaching*. 2nd edn. London: RoutledgeFalmer; 2002.

12 http://en.wikipedia.org/wiki/Netiquette

13 Draper S. *Interactive Lectures*. 2005. www.psy.gla.ac.uk/~steve/ilig/il.html

14 Bruff D. *Teaching with Classroom Response Systems: creating active learning environments*. San Francisco, CA: Jossey-Bass; 2009.

15 www.keele.org.uk/cubes

16 www.plagiarismadvice.org/resources/designing-out-plagiarism

17 www.submit.ac.uk

18 Bostock SJ. Motivation and electronic assessment. In: Irons A, Alexander S, eds. *Effective Learning and Teaching in Computing*. London: RoutledgeFalmer; 2004. pp. 86–99.

FURTHER READING

• Bostock SJ. *e-Teaching: engaging learners through technology*. London: Staff and Educational Development Association; 2007.

• Essential Skills in Technology Enhanced Medical Education (ESTEME). www.amee.org/index.asp?lm=97

• International Virtual Medical School (IVIMEDS). www.ivimeds.org

CHAPTER 10

Teaching in ambulatory care settings

Helen Batty

REALISTIC SETTINGS FOR LEARNING

Previously, clinical training mainly took place in hospitals – on wards, in operating theatres and as part of outpatient department visits. Increasingly, however, patient care is now moving into the community and patients' own homes. Therefore more clinical teaching needs to happen there, too.[1,2] This can be an unwelcome challenge for teachers who are used to the relatively more predictable and well-structured hospital environment.

Learners in all healthcare disciplines will benefit from educational experiences with ambulatory patients in settings that truly reflect the context that will comprise these learners' own future practices. It is easier for learners to remember knowledge, skills and attitudes when they are recalled in the same context as that in which they were learned.

Opportunities for learners to work in a variety of settings away from the wards, starting early in their professional training, also help them to understand the variety of career options and styles of practice available to them in their own futures. Most patients are 'ambulatory', arriving at our clinical locations for only a few minutes or hours. Seeing patients in their own homes and in community settings accurately demonstrates the environments to which hospital patients are returning after discharge, and the resources that are available (or not) to enhance their treatment and care.

TEACHING THE IMPORTANCE OF TEAMWORK

Teamwork is crucial for effective, safe and cost-efficient healthcare outside the hospital, especially for patients with complex or chronic serious illnesses. Preparing learners to practise in teams and in these difficult ambulatory situations by introducing them early and supporting their growing involvement is essential for building their confidence and competence.

The *communities of practice* theory[3] states that well-functioning teams grow together over time and develop new knowledge, protocols and supportive networks. This allows teams to improve the care of their specific community of patients. Therefore it is very important that team function is understood and valued by teachers and learners. Informally, learners can be 'legitimate peripheral observers' watching from the edge of a team function or meeting. As the learners' time and experience with the team increase, teachers should highlight opportunities when learners can take a more active role within the team and in team meetings (e.g. making a case presentation for team discussion, or undertaking a literature search for information required by the team).

Learning the manners, etiquette, courtesies and nuances of team cooperation and communication are vital competences for healthcare professionals. Helping learners to appreciate teamwork and to feel supported to participate in healthcare teams is a major role for teachers.

Teamwork takes time. Teachers and learners need protected time away from direct patient care to discuss cases with other team members informally or at formal team meetings. Initially this may feel as if the patients are being disadvantaged. However, in the long run, patients who are being cared for by a well-functioning team will have a greater proportion of their care attended to more efficiently, particularly if they have complex or chronic illnesses.

When learners are at an early stage of developing confidence in patient interviewing and physical examination, the teacher needs to balance this important practice time with their need to also learn about being part of a team for the reasons highlighted above.

TECHNOLOGY IN THE AMBULATORY CARE SETTING
Technological tools

Telephones, fax machines, computers, video recordings, the Internet, etc. are all used to support patient care, communication, and cooperation among team members and with patients and families, referral consultants and hospitals, community resources and other institutions. They are integral for learners to also see and use themselves.

Applications of technology

➤ Communication – between and among healthcare professionals and patients.
➤ Health information:
— storage and management of patient records (in electronic medical records)
— quality of care assurance (conducting surveys, chart audits, etc.).
➤ Knowledge acquisition by:
— health practitioners
— patients and families.

Learners should not spend all of their time undertaking direct patient contact. They will benefit from spending some time at workstations or talking on the telephone, both of which are essential elements of healthcare practice. Supervise this activity to help learners to become time-efficient, follow appropriate professional protocols and display appropriate attitudes.

Educational technology is helpful for:
➤ monitoring or assessment of learners
➤ observation of or reflection on clinical work
➤ structured teaching modules/'learning objects'
➤ simulation of complex or new practical skills or teamwork situations

➤ distance transmission and reception (teleconferencing audio-only or audio-visual of lectures, seminars, discussions or other educational activities from a remote programme base site).

Tips from experienced teachers

- A single phone line can provide effective distance education if linked to a fax machine to receive graphics (diagrams, pictures, etc.) and text in advance of a session, plus a standard telephone receiver or speaker phone so that one or more people can listen and discuss the topic in real time either one to one with a teacher, or as part of a small group.
- Observing students' work in person is easier if you explain to the patient what the intention is (e.g. 'I am supervising this learner and I would like to watch them in action to help with their training'). You should look intently at the learner rather than looking at, or responding to, visual cues from the patient.
- During direct observation of a learner from another room, you could telephone the learner briefly to make recommendations or suggest that the learner comes and speaks privately with you.

AREAS THAT REQUIRE EXTRA ATTENTION

Many aspects of clinical teaching 'away from the ward' require extra thought and effort, particularly when there is less traditional routine or established structure to rely upon.

Getting yourself ready

If you are teaching a programme for the first time, or if the curriculum has been newly revised, make sure that you read all of the available documentation, learning objectives, outlines, forms requiring completion, etc., well in advance. Check to see whether the programme has any faculty development sessions available to acquaint you with their expectations and usual teaching methods. If you have questions or concerns, discuss them with the programme director ahead of time.

Before the learner arrives

Identify where the learner will be able to:
➤ securely leave their personal belongings
➤ observe and talk with team members
➤ take a break or use toilet facilities
➤ interview and examine patients privately
➤ discuss quick questions with you
➤ sit with you for a full case discussion
➤ write information in the patient's notes.

Also decide where you can observe the learner.

Other team members

Your team members must be involved in discussions before you agree to accept a learner into your clinical setting.

This discussion should include issues relating to the following.

➤ Who is responsible for the learner's clinical work?

➤ Who will supervise the learner?

➤ Who is providing informal feedback and formal assessment?

➤ Acknowledgment that the presence of a learner will add complexity and reduce efficiency for the whole team

➤ Is any remuneration or reward available to the team as a whole in some form, or to individual team members?

Some teams may also want to ensure that no one health profession is favoured. Without clear and appropriate reasons, there should be no assignment of learners from one particular health profession to the team over acceptance of learners from other health professions.

Patients and their families

There must be full awareness and disclosure when a clinical setting or healthcare team is part of an educational programme. This is easy if teaching starts at the same time as the clinic is established or the teams form. However, when teaching responsibilities are added into pre-existing healthcare settings, there must be careful preparation for the clients or patients. Giving advance notice by verbal explanation and/or by posting signs in waiting-room areas works well.

Patients and their families must always, whenever appropriate, be allowed to refuse to have a learner present during their care. Talking to patients in advance may help to introduce the idea of including a learner, or actually introducing the learner in person may win agreement for the learner to be involved.

Patients and families can often feel that they are making a significant contribution to improving the healthcare system for themselves and others in the future when they allow a learner to be part of their encounter and ongoing relationship with the health-care team. Such patients may even agree to schedule sessions at times when teaching is required.

Tips from experienced teachers

- Patients who are healthcare professionals, teachers in other topic areas or whose families have benefited from effective healthcare (or occasionally suffered unfortunate adverse experiences in the healthcare system) may be eager to help you and your team in training future healthcare professionals. Never be afraid to ask patients to volunteer to be included in your teaching team.
- The more time you spend appropriately orientating a learner, the more efficient your subsequent teaching and their clinical work will be.
- You can learn a lot from your learners, sometimes in unexpected ways.

Appropriate learning resources

Everything that the learner sees, hears, smells, touches and feels in your clinical set-ting adds to their education experience. Capitalise on these opportunities by taking a broad view of what is happening from minute to minute. Introduce this concept to the learner at the beginning of your orientation, and ask the learner to communicate what they are noticing or wondering about while they are with you. Help them to reflect on it.

Learners benefit from many of the information sources that are available in any healthcare setting. Encourage them to review whatever paperwork is completed or given to patients and their families. Similarly, make sure that they are aware of the forms, guidelines, brochures, booklets and other hard copies that team members share. Show them whatever reference resources you use, and suggest that they begin to build their own selection of resources. Watch to see what they are using to solve clinical problems while they are with you.

ORIENTATION: INTRODUCING THE LEARNER

Once your clinical setting and team are ready to receive learners, plan how you will orientate them.

Introduce all learning resources to the learner as early as possible. Useful information could be written in a letter or memo to be given to the learner on the first day or sent in advance. Generally, the longer you expect a learner to be with you, the more extensive an orientation you should organise. For example, you might spend two weeks orientating a learner who will be training with you for two years.

You can select appropriate patients and clinical tasks by checking in advance the list of cases scheduled for a teaching session. 'Prime' the learner about patients before they see them. Provide a quick synopsis and advise them of the task or area on which to focus. Also prepare learners if you anticipate any difficulties.

During your first sessions with a new learner, consider allowing them to observe you. Role modelling is an efficient way to show what is possible, appropriate and expected from them. Demonstrate a variety of activities to provide a full picture – interviewing and examining patients, discussions with the team, and managing paperwork and telephone calls. For novice learners, start by highlighting basic aspects of what you are doing. For more advanced learners, use this as an opportunity to share subtle techniques and fine points and receive helpful comments from them.

APPROPRIATE MONITORING OF LEARNERS' ACTIVITIES
Direct observation

You may be supervising a situation where neither the learner nor the patient is known to you. This can be stressful, as you hold full responsibility for the clinical care of the patient. If you are in doubt about the learner's level of competence, directly observe the clinical encounter. Once you are confident in the learner's growing abilities, you can reduce the amount and intensity of direct supervision.

Watching the learner work while you are in the room, or remotely using video/web cams and microphones, is the most accurate way to gauge their confidence and competence. With novice learners, focus on only one aspect of the clinical encounter – perhaps the part that seems most appropriate or the main priority (e.g. physical examination, the closing summary). Discuss and agree with the learner in advance what you plan to focus on. Avoid overloading yourself, the learner or the patient. In all cases, the camera is focused primarily on the learner. Cameras should be turned off when a patient disrobes or is in the room without the learner. You must have appropriate patient consent prior to activating any such system.

Generally, you should try not to interrupt the learner once they have started. However, occasionally you may be concerned enough to take over and finish the patient encounter. If this happens you could:

➤ consider moving away from the patient briefly to discuss the case, and advise the learner that you will take charge of the situation when you both return

➤ make a gentle but direct comment to the learner suggesting that, given the available time, you recommend switching places so that the patient can be appropriately accommodated

➤ suggest that the learner moves to another task, such as looking up laboratory results, taking a message to another team member or consulting the literature, while you expeditiously proceed with the care of the patient.

Indirect supervision

Depending on your setting and the level of your learner, you may wish to regularly review what the learner is doing during a session and before the patient leaves. With novice learners, you can request that they come to you after interviewing a patient to discuss the information that they have acquired, before and after any physical examination, before finalising a treatment plan and before sending the patient away or finishing the visit. For senior learners, you may be happy that they work at an efficient pace throughout the whole session and come to you only with occasional urgent questions. At the end of either situation discuss the highlights of the cases that they have seen, and arrange a final sign-off.

Tips from experienced teachers

- If you are simultaneously trying to undertake clinical work of your own while teaching others, you must clearly give learners permission to interrupt your work at any time if they need your advice. You should remain close at hand.
- Many teachers in the ambulatory clinical session find the 'One Minute Preceptor' a helpful framework for time-effective teaching and giving feedback (*see* Chapter 8).
- If you are short of time to give feedback to learners, share the positive feedback publically and write any specific suggestions for change in a private hard-copy message, with an invitation to the learner to contact you later for further discussion if they wish.

Keeping alert to cues that a learner might be struggling is an important skill for a teacher in an ambulatory care setting to develop.

Signs that the learner is struggling

➤ Taking an unusually long time with the patient.

➤ Coming to you with unexpected concerns about a patient.

➤ Behaviour that is out of character for that particular learner (they may be mimicking the patient's behaviour unconsciously – confusion or hypomania can be contagious).

➤ Bringing a disorganised description of the history or examination that they have just completed.

➤ The learner discussing the case with another health professional when you are available to review the clinical work.

CONCLUDING A TEACHING SESSION

Arrange a final summative 'sit-down' group review of all the cases seen in the session before everyone leaves. Involving learners at a variety of levels and other team members can be very beneficial.

Ask the members of the group to take turns to summarise and highlight each case individually to stimulate reflection, or discuss the most interesting or unusual cases or a particular clinical theme that has emerged. For example, you may have noticed that a number of similar cases seem to be related to a particular virus. You could facilitate a shared discussion about the aspects and implications of this infection currently prevalent in your community.

FEEDBACK: FORMATIVE DISCUSSION

Learners highly value constructive comments about their work. They may not feel confident about asking you directly, so consciously plan to offer generous, honest, positive reinforcement of their correct actions and strong qualities. Suggestions for improvement may be given in small, careful doses throughout any teaching session (*see* Chapter 13 for information on providing effective feedback).

In an ambulatory care setting you may only be working with learners briefly, so provide succinct feedback with every case, at the halfway point of any teaching session and before you part each day. If you have the opportunity to work with a learner for more than one session, arrange with them in advance how any topics that have been discussed will be monitored in future sessions. You must have some follow-up on actions agreed to or discussed.

FOSTERING INDEPENDENCE

Encouraging increasingly independent practice, self-directed learning and team-based continuing professional development are all valuable lessons for learners in an ambulatory care setting. Learners must experience taking responsibility, problem solving and working with other healthcare team members. The longer you are working with a learner, the easier it will be for you to judge how much independence they can be granted. Initially, assign learners very specific small tasks to determine how much they can handle. Ask them what they feel they are prepared for and what they would like to do in each case. Obtain the opinions of other members of your healthcare team about learners' levels of competence.

If you have several learners simultaneously, encourage them to interact, teach and help each other. Advanced learners can share your supervision of a novice learner. In return, you should provide extra stimulation and intellectual challenge to the senior learners.

ASSESSMENT: SUMMATIVE EVALUATION REPORTS

You may be required to assess learners (*see* Chapter 14). Ambulatory teaching provides the opportunity to make a particularly accurate assessment of a learner's capabilities, as it is a realistic setting. Often learners have not previously had a chance to build an ongoing relationship with a teacher who can assess them as individually as this.

Tips from experienced teachers

- Keep brief 'field notes' for each teaching session, just as you would for clinical case work.
- If unexpected difficulties arise:
  - ask a team member or senior learner to work with or directly teach the learner
  - tell the learner to continue with you at their side for support
  - speak privately with the person to obtain more understanding of the situation
  - take over and role model appropriate actions.
- A teaching session with too few patients can provide the opportunity to role model making good use of time in your management of paperwork, attending to other team responsibilities, and following up unanswered questions or interesting cases.
- A session in which you are feeling overwhelmed with patient problems is an excellent time to teach about maintaining professional composure, setting priorities, delegating responsibility and working with patients' and families' prime concerns.

As assessments can be major turning points in a learner's career, you must find out *before* the learner arrives exactly what kind of assessment is expected. Clarify any uncertainties about programme expectations or assessments with the authorities who are responsible for the learner well in advance.

DEVELOPING TEACHING STRATEGIES FOR UNEXPECTED SITUATIONS AND ADAPTING TO AMBULATORY SETTINGS

Boxes 10.1 and 10.2 list the advantages and disadvantages of teaching in ambulatory settings.

BOX 10.1 Advantages of ambulatory teaching

- Builds a meaningful one-to-one relationship with learners.
- Enables clinical experience to be tailored to individual learner needs.
- Stimulating for the team.
- Educational for the teacher.
- Patients derive satisfaction from contributing to education of healthcare professionals.
- Perceptive learners bring new ideas to the clinical setting on many levels.
- The learner's experience is aligned with the needs of their own real-world future practice.

BOX 10.2 Disadvantages of ambulatory teaching

- Adds another layer of unpredictability for the clinical team.
- Results in extra responsibility and work for the clinician teacher.
- Time-stressed environment.
- Potentially chaotic clinical setting.
- Unhappy patients and families.
- Reduced efficiency of care.

Things to do

By nature, you cannot specifically prepare for unexpected events. However, you can prepare to manage unexpected circumstances to the best of your abilities.

➤ Expect the unexpected.
➤ Take a moment to consider the situation.
➤ Trust your first instinct.
➤ Ask the learner for ideas.
➤ Ask your team for ideas.
➤ Ask the patient and their family for ideas.
➤ Limit yourself to only highlighting one teaching point per case.
➤ Focus on a positive aspect of the situation.
➤ Debrief afterwards with the learners, discussing your reflections on aspects of the process or content that surprised you.
➤ Explore what other teachers do by attending education conferences, reading about teaching, and encouraging discussion among your colleagues.

Things that can go wrong

Things that can go wrong in the ambulatory setting include the following.

➤ No patients are available.
➤ Patients refuse to see or speak with a learner.
➤ A patient requires emergency treatment and urgent transfer to a hospital setting.
➤ Too many patients have been booked for the number of learners scheduled.
➤ The learner refuses to see a particular patient or follow your treatment recommendations.
➤ A patient's accompanying family or companion, the team or you are distressed.

SPECIAL THINGS TO REMEMBER ABOUT HOME/COMMUNITY VISITS

➤ You are guests in the setting.
➤ It will take extra time initially to acknowledge the people present and their context.
➤ Be prepared to leave at any time if requested to do so.
➤ Social conventions may require you to drink, eat, look at photographs, admire special objects and otherwise become involved with your patient and their life. Take advantage of the opportunity to make observations about aspects of the patient and the situation which you have not previously considered.

➤ Establishing appropriate professional boundaries can be challenging, but this is an ideal opportunity for learners to gain practice in doing so.
➤ Travelling together may give you and the learners an excellent opportunity for conversation about the particular case, general education issues or broad philosophical ideas.

TIME MANAGEMENT

The challenge is to find an efficient balance of good patient care with meaningful contributions to learners' education experience. There are a number of things you can do to manage time effectively.

➤ Accomplish your most difficult teaching task at the beginning of any session.
➤ Focus on the learners' identified interests.
➤ Choose one small but significant teaching point per case.
➤ Avoid 'over-teaching.' Conserve your strength and don't talk too much.
➤ Check with the learner halfway through the session for adjustments of your initial time management plan.
➤ Rescue any learner who appears to be flagging – offer them a break or change of activity.
➤ Find opportunities to enable senior learners to become part of your teaching team.
➤ Listen to any immediate scheduling concerns that team members bring to you.
➤ Encourage all team members to watch for and act upon ways to improve educational efficiencies minute by minute.
➤ Monitor your own energy level and plan accordingly.
➤ Advise the learners and team of any unusual time constraints at the beginning of the session.
➤ Plan to end the session with a teaching activity which you and the learners look forward to.

REFERENCES

1 Dent JA. AMEE Guide No 26. Clinical teaching in ambulatory care settings: making the most of learning opportunities with outpatients. *Med Teacher.* 2005; **27**: 302–15.
2 Irby DM, Bowen JL. Time-efficient strategies for learning and performance. *Clin Teacher.* 2004; **1**: 23–8.
3 Wenger E. *Communities of Practice: learning, meaning and identity.* Cambridge: Cambridge University Press; 1998.

FURTHER READING

• Wenger E. *Communities of Practice: a brief introduction.* www.ewenger.com/theory/index. htm
• Rubinstein W, Talbot Y. *Medical Teaching in Ambulatory Care.* 2nd edn. New York: Springer Publishing Company; 2003.

CHAPTER 11

Organising educational activities

Good organisation and preparation are key to obtaining maximum benefit from any educational activity. You have a duty of care to ensure that learners will not be wasting time by attending the activity. Not only should you provide quality education, but you should also ensure that everything runs smoothly and nothing is left to chance. This chapter covers practical tips that you will want to take into account when organising a meeting of any size, or a course.

ORGANISING A MEETING

If you are too busy to organise an event, you could employ a commercial conference organiser. They may organise the entire event at no cost to you, but will arrange and retain a proportion of sponsorship and delegates' fees.

You cannot fail to organise a successful meeting or conference if you choose a subject that addresses people's needs, at a price they can afford, at a convenient time in an accessible location. A subject that is both topical and new to a wide range of healthcare professionals and managers will maximise the number of potential delegates.

Select and book the venue

To minimise the risk of things going wrong (*see* Box 11.1), choose a central location to which people can easily travel. If it is a regional or national event, ensure proximity to a major train station and easy access to motorways. If it is a local event, ensure that car parking is relatively easy. If the meeting is being held after normal working hours, the venue should be well lit and secure. Consider whether there is to be small group work (for which you need plenty of separate break-out rooms), and take into account the expected number of delegates when deciding on the size and number of rooms needed.

BOX 11.1 Things that can go wrong when organising educational events
- Too few delegates register so
  - the event is not viable and has to be cancelled
  - you run the event at a financial loss.
- Speakers don't turn up.
- Delegates arrive late because of travel problems.
- You overwork the delegates and deprive them of any opportunity to take advantage of their surroundings, despite having chosen the venue for its sporting facilities or rural situation.
- Paperwork is circulated to the delegates after the event because handouts were not available on time.
- Speakers are booked for their availability rather than their suitability for the task.
- You run a course or conference to fulfil your own educational needs or preferences rather than those of the intended audience.
- You choose an inappropriate teaching format due to organisational ease rather than it being the most suitable delivery method.

Cost different venues and research the catering arrangements. Some venues allow outside caterers to be used, while others insist that you use theirs at fixed (and often inflated) prices. Visit the venue if possible before booking it, especially if you are arranging a large or important conference. Its availability may indicate that it is noisy, draughty or cold. Book the caterer or meal and refreshments required.

Establish the availability of audiovisual equipment before making your booking. Organisation will be easier if you find a venue that supplies whatever technology is required for the presentations. Find out whether you have to pay extra for audiovisual equipment. Some venues charge for the hire of a flipchart or microphone, and this soon adds up, making venue costs higher than they initially seemed.

Estimate the approximate number of delegates that you expect. If you are paying the venue per delegate, err on the low side. You can always increase the numbers nearer to the event, and you may be charged extra if fewer delegates attend than anticipated. Arrange to confirm the exact numbers a few days prior to the meeting. Return the booking form, and note the date of cancellation after which financial penalties will be incurred.

Many venues insist that you pay a deposit, some or all of which may be forfeited if you cancel the conference, with a sliding scale depending on how long before the event the cancellation is made. Unless you are absolutely sure that you will hold the event no matter how few people attend, opt for a low-cost venue such as a postgraduate centre, rather than a plush hotel or conference centre. There is more chance that the manager will be understanding and tolerant of last-minute cancellations, and not insist on a financial penalty.

Prepare your budget

Estimate your costs and profit margin. Include the following:
➤ hire and costs of the venue
➤ the cost of food and drink – drinks priced per head can soon add up

➤ speakers' fees and travel or hotel expenses
➤ your time for organising/chairing the meeting
➤ any application fee for educational accreditation or other continuing medical education
➤ the cost of postage, advertisements, printing flyers, copying handouts or other course materials, stationery and administration
➤ delegates' fees – ensure that these cover costs for a minimum number of delegates and the amount of profit that you want to make. Allow for reimbursement of delegates' fees if they do not attend
➤ how much sponsorship you want – find generous commercial representatives whose products are relevant to the topic of your meeting.

Decide the programme

Check that no similar meetings which may be competing for the same audience are planned in your locality, or nationally if you are organising a big event.

Ensure that the programme is balanced and not overcrowded. Choose an appropriate mix of lectures, small group work and refreshment breaks, depending on the learning objectives for the meeting, the topic, the type of delegates, their likely attention span and the expertise of the speakers.

Think about the marketability of the programme. There is no point in arranging a very worthy meeting that no one wants to attend, unless there is a large pool of people who are compelled to attend in order to fulfil a legal or organisational requirement. You may have to sandwich topics that are less popular but very important with more light-hearted sessions to increase (continuing) attendance.

Choose start times that allow for travel to the venue. Finish at a convenient time if your audience is likely to need to pick up children from school or run an evening surgery or clinic. Don't face delegates with too long a programme – leave them wanting a little more.

Include sufficient time in the programme (e.g. by arranging a midday start, long lunch breaks, time off in the evening) for delegates to sample the facilities when appropriate. Don't encourage them to play truant to enjoy their surroundings.

Book your speakers

Telephone potential speakers to check their availability and issue a personal invitation. Follow this with a confirmatory letter giving full details of the meeting. The letter should include the following details:
➤ the date and time of the meeting
➤ the venue
➤ the expected audience
➤ the suggested title
➤ the angle and content you would like to have covered (unless you want to leave it open to them)
➤ the fee
➤ whether reimbursable expenses include accommodation, first-/second-class travel, etc.
➤ the response deadline.

Arrange postgraduate or continuing professional education accreditation

Once you have fixed the date, venue, programme and speakers, find out the requirements of all the professional organisations to which delegates are affiliated, and apply for approval for the relevant postgraduate or continuing medical educational accreditation in good time. It can take weeks for the paperwork to be processed.

Advertise the meeting

How can you best reach the delegates whom you hope will attend? For local events, circulate flyers around the hospital, universities, clinics or general practices. For regional or national events, place adverts in professional journals or newsletters that your target audience is likely to read. Reduce the costs of advertising by linking with someone else who is sending out material. Consider writing a short article about the meeting which will be placed as a free news item in newsletters or journals. Post flyers about your meeting on all the professional or public noticeboards you can possibly use. Leave piles of flyers at local meeting places or other similar educational meetings where delegates are likely to be interested in your event, too.

Your flyers should be eye-catching. Choose colour, an unusual design, a different shape, etc. to attract attention. Include all of the details that people need to enable them to book for the meeting. This includes the time, date, venue and location, the organisation, institution, etc. to whom cheques should be made payable, the type and amount of educational accreditation applied for, the programme outline, a description of the speakers and the target audience. Include an email address and telephone and fax numbers that will be responded to by someone who is familiar with the meeting and who will take responsibility for dealing with enquiries.

A few weeks before the meeting

Confirm the delegates' places, and if it is not a local event, send out a map of the venue as applications come in. Itemise cheques so that you know who has paid. Don't pay cheques into the bank until after the meeting if possible, in case the meeting is cancelled or you need to reimburse a delegate who cannot attend.

Contact the speakers again to remind them of their engagement, and answer any queries. Ascertain their audiovisual equipment requirements, encourage them to provide handouts, and obtain a short biography to enable a proper introduction. Send them a map of the location.

Circulate to the delegates any homework that is required in preparation for the meeting, with clear instructions for returning any work that needs to be assessed prior to the meeting, or any information that is needed to prime one of the speakers.

A few days before the meeting

Prepare an attendance list, evaluation forms, name badges and certificates to provide evidence of attendance. Name badge text should be large enough to be easily read at a distance of a metre. Consider including some information about where delegates originate from, but ensure that it is correct.

If appropriate, buy and wrap a present for a speaker or chair who is not charging a fee.

Book tables and boards outside the meeting room for sponsors or delegates who want to display goods or posters. Pack Velcro pads or Blu-Tack® for hanging posters.

Chase up speakers who have agreed to send in handouts. Copy sufficient numbers of handouts in advance of the event.

If you prepare well (*see* Boxes 11.2, 11.3 and 11.4), the meeting will be a success.

BOX 11.2 Key points to be considered when preparing
for the meeting or conference

- Find an appropriate and accessible venue.
- Make the catering arrangements.
- Calculate your budget and any delegates' fees.
- Seek sponsorship as necessary.
- Invite speakers, and confirm their terms and conditions.
- Finalise the programme.
- Apply for approval for educational accreditation.
- Advertise the meeting widely to groups that are likely to be interested.
- Confirm applicants' places and send out maps.
- Prepare paperwork for the meeting well in advance.
- Confirm the last-minute details with speakers.
- Obtain speakers' biographies.
- Encourage speakers to prepare handouts.

BOX 11.3 What to do at the meeting: key points

- Encourage the wearing of name badges.
- Check lighting and audiovisual equipment.
- Put the speakers at ease and in control.
- Sign the facilities well.
- Look after sponsors.
- Arrange speedy access to food and drinks.
- Encourage the completion of evaluation forms.
- Distribute handouts.

BOX 11.4 What to do after the meeting: key points

- Summarise the delegates' evaluations.
- Consider future educational events in the light of feedback.
- Write to thank the speakers, and feed back relevant evaluation as appropriate.
- Arrange for the speakers' fees to be paid.
- Check and pay the bills for the venue and catering.
- Prepare the final budget – profits or losses.
- Write and disseminate a report of the event as appropriate.

On the day of the meeting

Allow plenty of time for travel to the venue, to ensure that you arrive first. Don't dash in at the last minute and expect to impose order on speakers and delegates who are already milling around.

Critically view the venue and decide where is the best place to display notices to direct delegates to the meeting rooms. Signpost the toilets, and if these are limited near the main meeting room, indicate the way to additional toilets.

Organise refreshments so that delegates have several points of access to drinks to prevent long queues building up. Set up a registration desk for enrolling delegates and giving out programmes or instructions for the day. Ensure that sponsors have the display space they need in prominent positions, and enough to eat and drink.

Check that the audiovisual equipment is working. Arrange for a technician who services the audiovisual equipment or a porter to be available in case any problems occur with the equipment.

Arrange for a lapel microphone if the speaker wants to use an overhead projector or walk about. Organise a roving microphone to be available for questions from large audiences.

Brief the chairperson with the speakers' biographies, and check that the details are up to date. Introduce the speakers to the chairperson so that they can establish a rapport and understanding about the timing of the presentations.

Announce organisational details about fire exits, hospitality and refreshments, the location of toilets, and attendance and evaluation forms before the meeting and presentations begin. Include evaluation forms in the delegate's pack, or distribute them at the final tea break to promote completion.

Look after the speakers as they arrive. Find a quiet room for them if they want to practise their presentation or think through their talk. Ensure that fresh water is available when they speak. Show the speakers how to operate the audiovisual equipment and lighting, and offer help as necessary.

Ask the speakers for all of the details if you need to organise payment. Some speakers will require payment to be made to their employer, while others will want direct payment.

Relieve speakers of their handouts and arrange them on a table near an exit so that delegates can take what they want. Make extra copies before the event if there are not enough.

Organise a professional photographer or take pictures yourself of the audience or of any well-known speakers when the meeting is in full swing, for use in future marketing material.

Keeping to time – this is essential

Agree timings with the chairperson and the speaker(s), and a system for alerting them if they (nearly) overrun – for example, a hand signal, a bell or a coloured card. Insist that the chairperson and the speakers leave enough time for audience questions. If there is any doubt about whether everyone has heard all of the questions or comments, ask the chairperson to repeat what has been said before the speaker answers.

After the meeting

Collect the evaluation forms and summarise the contents. Send a copy to the unit responsible for accrediting the educational event if required. Feed back relevant remarks to speakers or the venue hosts. Consider a follow-up conference or meeting, depending on the delegates' feedback. Make a special note of positive comments to use in the advertising literature of any appropriate future events.

Write and thank the speakers and the chair, and arrange for their fees to be paid. Check the invoice from the venue carefully to see that the number of delegates and any extra services have been billed correctly before approving payment.

Consider writing a report of the meeting for wide dissemination of learning points or outcomes.

ORGANISING A COURSE

Day-to-day organisation of a course will follow the tips already described for organising individual events. However, additional considerations are introduced by the nature of the successive meetings of a course, often with self-directed work in between.

➤ Anticipate the need for participants to 'prove' the learning that they have experienced. Course programmes should provide the learning 'outcomes' and details of how evidence will be presented to prove that the set objectives have been addressed, reflection has taken place and outcomes have been achieved.

➤ The course coordinator should ensure the smooth running of the course, and that the right people and resources are in place at all the right times.

➤ A course tutor should support students who are in difficulty via email, telephone or face to face.

➤ Make it clear in the course details where the student can obtain necessary information about the course topics.

➤ Consider whether it is better for learners to attend teaching blocks of several whole days, or whether many weeks of short, part-day sessions are most appropriate. Long-distance learning courses offer an option in which learners can study at a time that is convenient to them.

Tips from experienced teachers

Key points for a successful meeting are as follows.
• Address people's learning and service needs.
• Set fees at reasonable cost.
• Choose an accessible location.
• Choose convenient timing.
• Avoid peak holiday times.
• Invite good speakers.
• Make the meeting interactive (active rather than passive learning).

FURTHER READING

• Knowles MS. *Androgogy in Action: applying modern principles of adult learning*. San Francisco, CA: Jossey-Bass; 1984.
• Pace CR. *College and University Environmental Scales: technical manual*. Princeton, NJ: Education Testing Service; 1963.

CHAPTER 12

Writing educational materials

Writing educational materials is a crucial teaching skill. Providing written information that is easy to use and well presented shows respect for learners. Don't skip this section because you have no intention of becoming an author of course materials, or writing a book or an article for a journal. Everyone who is involved in education should at least write programme details or information sheets (e.g. handouts for presentations or courses, or patient information about clinical procedures or situations). This chapter highlights the necessary considerations when writing educational materials.

USES OF EDUCATIONAL MATERIALS

The amount, type and format of information within educational materials will depend on the reason you are providing written materials. On the whole there are three main teacher-centred reasons:

1 to aid note-taking by providing a place for learners to make notes alongside an outline of the session, ensuring that they have all of the important information.
2 to provide extra detail or information that would detract from the flow of the lecture, but that learners need to make sense of what is being presented, such as reports, figures or tables
3 to provide extra information, such as vignettes for case discussion or small group work.

Learner-centred reasons for providing educational materials include the following:
➤ to provide an aide-mémoire, perhaps for revision for exams, of what was said, with personal annotations noting what was interesting or seemed important
➤ to provide a record of what was said, in order to:
— avoid note-taking and thus aid concentration
— replace missed teaching sessions.

Sometimes educational materials are given to learners after the event to assess what has been learned or to provide learners with information that was requested or noted to be missing within the teaching session.

Be clear about what you are trying to provide, to ensure that it will enhance your learners' education experience, rather than being a waste of time and resources.

CHOOSE THE FORMAT

Traditionally, written materials have been information sheets with bullet points or a printout of slides from a lecture. However, as technology progresses and becomes cheaper, you can choose to produce paper copies or electronic materials on CD, memory sticks, or via email or online learning environments (*see* Chapter 9). Before deciding which format to use, you need to consider your budget and the advantages and disadvantages of different options.

If you want to provide paper copies, think about how much information you want to distribute. One advantage of providing paper copies is that students can annotate the information provided with their own thoughts or quotes from the teacher. Some people find it much easier to read information on paper than on a computer screen. However, paper handouts can be messy, may become separated and are difficult to navigate, compared with electronic filing systems. Depending upon how much information you are providing, you may spend substantial time and money printing, collating and producing the handouts, particularly for large numbers of learners. Once it has been printed, written information cannot be altered or updated.

Electronic information is easier to navigate and takes up less physical space, as it can be saved on the learners' personal computers. People may therefore be more likely to keep the information. Updating or altering information remains an issue when using a CD, memory stick or email. However, providing additional materials in a virtual learning environment (*see* Chapter 9) overcomes this disadvantage. Providing electronic information often means that learners cannot immediately see what information they have been given, and so they may get distracted while taking notes on information that has been provided. It is also difficult for learners to annotate the information given.

PLAN THE CONTENT

Once you have decided on the aim and format, you need to start writing. First, plan an outline (*see* Box 12.1). Educational materials should capture the key points of your session, but need not be too comprehensive, as those who are particularly interested in the topic can follow up your session with private reading. Therefore further reading lists, references to key literature or details of additional information are useful inclusions. Educational materials do not have to be just a source of information, but can be used to assess prior knowledge and/or the extent of learning. Materials that include activities or interactivity (e.g. completing the blanks) can promote active learning.

BOX 12.1 Make an outline plan for your writing

- Introduction, to include definitions and objectives.
- Main themes: usually three, four or five.
- Discussion.
- Conclusions.
- Further ideas.
- References.
- Sources of further information.

You may find it difficult to start writing. Imagine a particular person you are writing for, and hold their image in your mind. Start with the section that interests you most and note your ideas. You can always write the introduction and link it into an expanded middle section later on. Let your writing flow without worrying too much about the phraseology or the grammar, which can be corrected when you refine your first draft. If you are unsure of spellings, use the spellchecker on your computer, but watch out for words that sound the same but are spelt differently (e.g. there and their), as these mistakes won't be detected.

Begin the piece by attracting the learner's attention with a clear, challenging statement, a rhetorical question, a short story or some other opening gambit. Where appropriate you could use alternative ways of communicating information. For example, 'graphic pathographies'[1] are graphic stories or 'illness narratives in graphic form.' Inclusion of such pictures could be enlightening to healthcare professionals, as such depictions of illness can provide new insights into patient experiences and misconceptions of illness, improve the learners' diagnostic skills and enhance their observational and interpretive abilities.[1] Pictures or cartoons can be included to inject fun and promote discussion in line with the theme of the session.[2]

Interest the reader by making it personally relevant for them. The use of 'you' rather than 'one' is more informal and involves the reader. Similarly, the use of plural pronouns (we, us, our) may appear less instructional and invites collaboration between teacher and learner.

When you are satisfied with your writing, ask someone else to read it through and comment on its readability and appropriateness for the target audience. This is particularly important if you are producing pre- or post-event assessments, as ambiguous questions are frustrating for learners.

The rules of copyright preclude you from photocopying large sections of published work for dissemination to students unless the publishers have printed their express permission for their work to be photocopied. This has implications if you are teaching critical reading skills and wish to provide copies of journals for the session. Handouts in advance of such a session could give the reference so that learners can bring the articles along themselves – and hopefully read it in preparation! You are usually allowed to copy about 5% of a literary work for your own research or private study. You may be able to obtain the author's or publisher's permission to provide photocopies of specific articles for learners if you write and ask them.

SUPPLYING EDUCATIONAL MATERIALS

The reasons for providing educational materials will govern not only what they contain but also when you give them out.

➤ If they are given out beforehand, this allows preparation or homework, can set the scene, allows problems to be identified, and enables learning at the session to build upon a common foundation of knowledge.
➤ If given out at the start of a session they can distract the audience, who may spend time reading them and not listening.
➤ If not given out until the end, they cannot be annotated and personalised, but . . .
➤ If not given out until the end, learners are 'persuaded' against leaving early.
➤ If they are given out at the start, time should be provided for learners to look at

and be aware of the content so that they will recognise new information in the lecture or associated discussion that might need to be noted down.

Tips from experienced teachers

- Write in clear, simple language.
- Use short sentences.
- Do not use two-syllable words if a one-syllable word will suffice.
- Pitch the content at the right level for the reader.
- Make the layout attractive, with plenty of white space.
- Include boxes for key points.
- Use subheadings to break up the text.
- Add illustrations and diagrams to complement the text.
- Focus on relevant material rather than rambling anecdotes.
- Explain any jargon or abbreviations.

Some learners need to know whether materials will be issued so that they can listen at a different level. Reflective learners may not concentrate on detail that they can read later, but on making internal maps and integrating this new information with what they already know.

REFERENCES

1 Green MJ, Myers KR. Graphic medicine: use of comics in medical education and patient care. *BMJ*. 2010; **340**: 574–7.
2 Chambers R, Wakley G, Iqbal Z *et al*. Written and audiovisual aids to learning. In: *Prescription for Learning: techniques, games and activities*. Oxford: Radcliffe Medical Press; 2002. pp. 229–35.

CHAPTER 13

Giving effective feedback

Constructive feedback is the art of holding conversations with learners about their performance, and has two elements. It should:
➤ contain enough specific detail and advice to enable the recipient to reflect and enhance their practice
➤ be positive and supportive in tone.

It is a very important concept in education, and can make or break any educational activity.

> Feedback, or knowledge of results, is the lifeblood of learning.[1]

Constructive feedback affects the teaching/learning process and informs learners about their effectiveness and worth. It has an indirect effect on their academic self-esteem.
This chapter presents:
➤ evidence that giving feedback effectively and positively, whether the content is praise or aspects that need to be improved, enhances learning
➤ simple methods and models for giving constructive feedback (i.e. giving suggestions for improvement without damaging morale).

Information on using information technology to provide feedback can be found in Chapter 9.

GOOD CLINICAL TEACHING: THE EVIDENCE
Concern about the standard of clinical teaching in UK hospitals has existed for some time.[2-4] Teaching by humiliation and ritual sarcasm, and the demotivating effects that this may have on trainees, has been described.[5] Similar problems exist in North America, where a literature review showed that undergraduate and postgraduate medical teaching was variable, unpredictable, lacked continuity and gave virtually no feedback.[6] In Australia, little feedback, poor supervision and haphazard assessment of junior doctors have also been described.[7]

Nursing and midwifery research throughout the 1990s also showed that feedback was handled poorly or, worse, was not carried out at all.[8] Consider the following quote from a nursing assessor:

> I shy away from having to give criticism. I'll always go to great lengths not to give criticism. . . . I'll always highlight the positive aspects and tend not to go into many details if the student isn't doing terribly well in certain areas.[8]

To address these issues and improve teaching and the educational climate in hospitals, the Standing Committee on Postgraduate Medical and Dental Education (SCOPME)[9] provoked professional debate about the need to improve clinical teaching.[10,11] Coles concluded that a change in educational and teaching methods, rather than a rearrangement of course content, was needed to enhance the teaching culture and give constructive feedback.[12]

Research has highlighted the importance of feedback being perceived as constructive. 'Giving feedback constructively' was the top theme chosen by 441 junior and senior doctors when asked what they thought should be the key content of 'Teaching the Teachers' courses.[13]

GIVING CONSTRUCTIVE FEEDBACK: SOME EVIDENCE THAT IT WORKS

Does it work? Is there evidence that giving constructive feedback improves learning? In short, the answer is yes. Constructive feedback can improve learning outcomes and enable learners to develop a deep (rather than superficial) approach to their learning with the active pursuit of understanding and application of knowledge. It can improve competence at least in the short term.[14] Giving constructive feedback does produce significantly better learning outcomes.[3]

WHAT TO AVOID IN FEEDBACK

Some teachers struggle to find the balance between giving 'feedback with teeth' – that is, feedback containing enough specific examples of where performance needs to be improved (sometimes, confusingly, called negative feedback) – and doing it in a negative or unhelpful way. You may hear teachers say that in a situation where time is short, it is better just to focus on aspects that the learner needs to improve on, without seeming to realise that this approach and being encouraging in tone are not mutually exclusive. Positive methods do have a better effect on the learner than negative methods.

Many well-trained teachers know the principles of giving constructive feedback. However, they may slip back into giving negative feedback, with disastrous results. Keep check of the feedback you give to ensure that this does not happen to you with your learners.

Recent guidance emphasises the importance of feedback in the teacher's role, but also highlights the fact that:

> performance cannot improve without knowledge of what was wrong, and there will come a time when it may be too late to give critical feedback – the learning opportunity may be lost and the behaviour entrenched.[15]

Some guidance for nurse educators, who generally tend to shy away from giving critical feedback, makes no mention of reinforcing good performance, perhaps making the assumption that this aspect is automatically well addressed. Nurse assessors are advised that the role of assessor requires a commitment to constructive feedback, and that it is the responsibility of the assessor to establish communication, clarify any problems and either get a commitment to change or offer a solution.[16]

CONSTRUCTIVE FEEDBACK

As well as being positive in tone, there should be a balance between comment on areas where improvement is needed and feedback that is positive in content. You should give feedback about deficiencies and strengths to assist your learners to develop expertise (*see* Figure 13.1).

Starting in the top left-hand quadrant in Figure 13.1, learners are blissfully unaware of their shortcomings until something happens to highlight them. It could be a patient complaint or an adverse incident, or it could be feedback from a teacher.

This realisation is painful, and is often referred to as cognitive dissonance. However, until learners are aware they cannot start the process of learning. Inform learners that often when they feel most uncomfortable they are just about to learn something. However, too much discomfort can be demotivating, and some learners might give up at this stage if they feel that there is too much to learn or that they will never be good enough. Providing feedback about their strengths will undoubtedly be supportive at this stage.

The process of learning can then proceed to master the new understanding, knowledge or task. The learner reaches a stage where they know something new or know how to do something and can competently perform it, so long as circumstances remain constant (*see* the bottom right quadrant of Figure 13.1). With practice and experience, learners become expert and can apply and modify their knowledge and skills in new situations. At this stage (bottom left quadrant), learners can teach others. It is also the stage when, through familiarity, learners can lose sight of their strengths, as skills

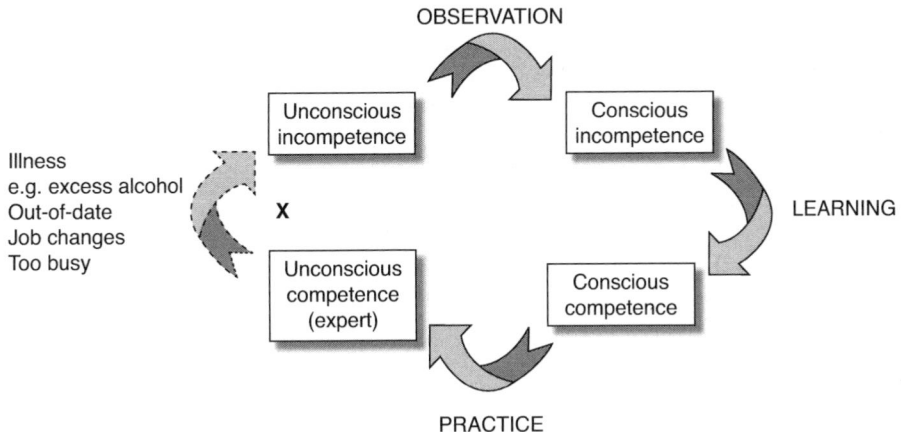

FIGURE 13.1

High support

'That was great, you're obviously trying hard.'	'A good effort. I could see how you were drawing the feelings out – I wonder if you got to the crux of the matter . . .?'
Safe, general, potentially patronising.	*Focused, attentive, potentially threatening.*
'Good. Carry on. Seems to be working.'	'Well that could have been better – why did you not focus more early on?'
In passing, nothing specific, dismissive.	*Critical – induces defensiveness, potentially paralysing.*

Low challenge (left) **High challenge** (right)

Low support

FIGURE 13.2

become automatic. Feedback on performance at this stage must include strengths, so that learners do not accept them as commonplace, and so that they reflect on them, keep them up to date and highlight them. In some ways, feedback should take learners from left to right across the bottom of the competency cycle to ensure that they are aware of their expertise, so that they can effectively teach others.

It is possible to move back to unconscious incompetence from the position of expertise, in the direction of arrow X, through, for example, dementing illness, degenerative disease without insight, and failure to keep up to date. Feedback in this position is difficult, which is another good reason to include a reminder of remaining skills and positive attributes. (This model has some similarities with the Johari window, which describes balanced communication between feedback seeking and self-disclosure to minimise either the areas of hidden information in a relationship or lack of insight; *see* Chapter 17.)

This model provides a theoretical reason why constructive feedback must contain a commentary on strengths as well as areas for improvement. It also reinforces the imperative for feedback to 'have teeth.' The skill of the effective teacher is to find the balance between support and challenge (*see* Figure 13.2). The best feedback is high in both.

METHODS OF GIVING CONSTRUCTIVE FEEDBACK

Table 13.1 shows some examples of giving feedback.

TABLE 13.1 Examples of feedback

Evaluative, interpretive or judgemental	Descriptive, sensory-based
The beginning was awful, you just seemed to ignore her	At the start you were looking at the notes, which prevented eye contact
The beginning was excellent, great stuff	At the beginning you gave her your full attention and never lost eye contact – your facial expression registered interest in what she was saying
It's no good getting embarrassed when patients talk about their sexual history	I noticed you were very flushed when she spoke about her husband's impotence, and you lost eye contact

Here are some rules to consider and some models of feedback that will help you to do this in a structured way. Four examples are given below, but you will be able to find or devise more. Just remember one golden rule – give positive praise for things that have been done well first. The four examples are:

➤ Pendleton's rules
➤ the SCOPME model for giving feedback
➤ the Chicago model
➤ the six-step problem-solving model.

Pendleton's rules[17]

This model provides a useful set of general principles to be used in giving feedback after all kinds of activities, including practical skills, consultations, case presentations, etc. It is a step-by-step model, in which each step is important and should be performed sequentially.

1 The learner performs the activity.
2 Questions are allowed only on points of clarification of fact.
3 The learner says what they thought was done well.
4 The teacher says what they thought was done well.
5 The learner says what was not done so well and could be improved upon.
6 The teacher says what was not done so well and makes suggestions for improvement with discussion in a supportive manner.

This is useful for formal situations, with learners who do not like feedback (e.g. those who are nervous), when the learner lacks insight and to encourage learners to identify the good points of their performance.

The SCOPME model[18]

This model is not the most simple and clear cut, but it does follow the same principles in order to give constructive feedback.

1 Listen to the learner.
2 Reflect back – for further clarification.
3 Support.
4 Counsel.

5 Treat information in confidence.
6 Inform – without censuring.
7 Judge constructively.
8 Identify educational needs.
9 Construct and negotiate achievable learning plans.

The Chicago model[19]

The 'Chicago' model is similar to the other models, but has the great advantage of starting with a reminder of the aims and objectives that the learner is supposed to be addressing. It has six steps.
1 Review the aims and objectives of the job at the start.
2 Give interim feedback of a positive nature.
3 Ask the learner to give their self-appraisal of their performance to you.
4 Give feedback focusing on behaviour rather than on personality (e.g. what actually happened, sticking to the facts, not your opinions).
5 Give specific examples to illustrate your views.
6 Suggest specific strategies for the learner to improve their performance.

A six-step problem-solving model

This model seeks agreement between two individuals to solve problems, agree goals, aims and objectives, and so on. It depends on negotiations between two people who come to an agreement at two stages in the model. The six steps are as follows.
1 Problem is presented.
2 Problem is discussed.
3 Problem is agreed.
4 Solution is proposed.
5 Solution is discussed.
6 Solution is agreed.

As well as agreeing educational aims at the beginning of a job, you may find other uses for this model. For example, when things have gone wrong it can help you to decide exactly why this happened and where the difficulty lies.

Feedback about unacceptable behaviour

If you need to give feedback to someone whose behaviour is completely unacceptable, there are ways of delivering the information and still maintaining a relationship that will enable you to continue to work together and support that learner.
Consider the following tips.
➤ Make sure that the person is in the right frame of mind to receive feedback (e.g. not tired after a night on-call) before you start.
➤ Use a wake-up, warning phrase.
➤ State very simply what is not right.
➤ Give an example, if necessary.
➤ Relax the tone to allow for a positive response (usually an offer to improve ensues).
➤ Respond to the offer positively, but define specific measurable outcomes.
➤ Do not be drawn into discussion on justification of behaviour or your right to judge.
➤ If there is complete rejection, seek help (e.g. from your peers or line manager).

The conversation might sound something like this one:

> Morning John, I hope the on-call was not too busy? I saw Mrs Smith yesterday, she said to thank you for those new tablets, and they've done her the world of good. . . . John, there is something very serious that I have to bring up in our session today . . . I am worried that you are drinking alcohol too heavily and I would like to talk about why that is. . . . Yesterday when we spoke after evening surgery I could smell alcohol on your breath, and you were slurring your words. I had the same impression at lunchtime the day before, but was not sure. . . . Is this something I can help you with? . . . I am glad you plan to cut down, how about if we agree that you will not drink during the working day, and not at all if you are on call? . . . I am afraid we cannot debate this, you need to address it or you will not be able to work here. . . . Then I must ask you to take a fortnight's leave until I can take advice from the deanery about this.

Or:

> I am afraid we cannot debate this, you need to address it or you will not be able to work here. . . . Excellent, let's have another chat about it on Thursday and we can see how it's going. In the mean time, shall we meet at lunchtime to look at that audit? It's coming on really well.

There is also the need to consider professional help here. This should be the general practitioner of the doctor concerned, and possibly a consultant in occupational medicine. You must not become your learners' medical practitioner.

MULTI-SOURCE FEEDBACK (MSF) (360 DEGREE ASSESSMENT)

What is multi-source feedback (MSF)? MSF asks several people *who know you* to rate certain defined behaviours and attitudes. Different people have different views, because they see you from a different perspective – your dog's perspective of you will probably be very different from that of your mother-in-law!

MSF is an accepted method of ensuring appropriate professional behaviours of doctors.[20] It is widely used in industry and in the healthcare sector,[20] and is a workplace-based assessment tool that is useful for assessing attitudes and behaviours, rather than clinical skills or knowledge. The purposes of MSF include developing insight into strengths and weaknesses, enhancing culture change, measuring the potential of individuals (for career progression or selection) and enhancing team effectiveness. Box 13.1 describes good practice in using MSF.

Often the principal purpose of MSF in healthcare is the identification of those who may have a problem with interpersonal communication (i.e. communication with patients and colleagues and working in teams). What happens next is of crucial importance. If the purpose is to take people out, then the diagnosis must be certain, and the tool that is used must be highly reliable and valid, and be able to withstand legal challenge. On the other hand, if the purpose is to provide skilled feedback to help people to improve their performance, to improve care of patients, to reduce disharmony and friction within a team, and to mollify upset staff and colleagues, those of us giving feedback must know how to do this.

BOX 13.1 Tips for developing and using MSF

1 Develop a positive culture.
2 Be clear about its purpose.
3 Clearly express desirable behaviours.
4 Keep the number of items to be scored few in number.
5 Keep the scale of the MSF tool simple and fit for purpose.
6 Use 10 or more raters.
7 Compare the results with self-assessment.
8 Train those who will be giving feedback.
9 Involve those who are being assessed.
10 Incorporate development within the organisation.

Who should assess? When assessing doctors in training, other doctors, senior nurses, midwives, peers, managers and secretaries are all able to assess these interpersonal communication and teamworking qualities.[21] However, senior doctors and senior nurses are better than junior doctors, managers and peers at detecting poor performance among doctors in training.[22]

What about self-assessment? A review of MSF by Wood *et al*[20] revealed that self-ratings tend to be higher than MSF ratings, especially for less highly rated individuals. This may be problematic, as some of these poorly performing individuals may not accept that they have a problem, and that there is a consequent need for change to more acceptable behaviours.

How many raters do you need? Worldwide studies indicate that 10 or 11 raters are required to achieve sufficient reliability to be able to act upon the results. Whatever the numbers stated, you should know this figure when using any MSF tool. You should be wary of using MSF tools which state that only four raters are needed to achieve sufficient reliability.

For any MSF tool you need descriptions of behaviours, not just a numerical score. The tool must allow raters to describe good and/or problematic behaviour. Numerical scores alone make it very difficult, if not impossible, to offer help, constructive feedback and behaviour modification to an acceptable level.

The assessment of foundation doctors (newly qualified junior doctors) in the UK is an example of MSF in practice. Team Assessment of Behaviours (TAB) is the preferred tool.[21,22] The structured questionnaire allows assessment across four domains:
1 maintaining trust and professional relationships with patients
2 verbal communication skills
3 teamworking
4 working with colleagues and accessibility.

It is used as a formative tool to help people to improve. However, it is also a summative tool, as an acceptable MSF is required for the doctor to be signed up as having successfully completed all competences for foundation training.

How should we give feedback – acting on MSF results?

Be positive and constructive. For most people, even those with problems, there will be some good comments. Detail what the desired behaviours are, and what you expect. Box 13.2 gives an example set of comments from a real MSF.

BOX 13.2 Maintaining trust/professional relationships with patients

He needs to take time to develop a good rapport with patients
Always polite and listens to patients
Poor listener – gives the impression he is not listening at times.
Takes time to communicate with patients' relatives, but often uses jargon few can understand.
Always polite and caring.
He has gained in confidence in recent months and has become more aware of the patients' needs, and spends time talking to them and trying hard to understand what the patients want – to understand the problem in simple terms.
Always polite, and treats both staff and patients with dignity.
I have been *****'s consultant for the last six months; I have tried hard to get him to interact with patients with a more caring attitude and behaviour. He is trying hard I think!
Good with patients, but some find the accent difficult. One patient commented that she needed an interpreter.

Verbal communication skills

Speaks with a heavy ******** accent – difficult for some to understand.
Good English sometimes – but speaks very quickly at times and difficult to understand.
Good communication skills at times – but not consistently.
Good English always – understandable when giving information.
Problems speaking to patients' relatives; speaks in tone and pace they find difficult to understand, and uses jargon.

The comments in Box 13.2 reveal problems both with communication with patients and in terms of being a poor listener, using jargon and speaking too quickly. However, there are good comments as well, and this learner seems to be trying hard to improve.

When giving feedback, sit down in private with your learner and show them the results. Use one of the models for giving constructive feedback (e.g. Pendleton's rules[17]). Using the example in Box 13.2, there are good points, such as being a caring doctor and making improvements, and these must come first. There are many areas for improvement, including speaking too quickly, using jargon, and the learner's accent. When discussing these areas, emphasise that much of this can be improved upon with good communication skills training and feedback. Explain how this may be accessed and how you will reassess the learner to measure their progress. Whatever you do, follow it up!

In another individual, accessibility was one of the problems (*see* Box 13.3). Comments included statements about being late, and being difficult to find when on call.

BOX 13.3 Accessibility

Sometimes difficult to find when on call.
Takes proper responsibility. Always willing to help when asked.
Always attentive to his job, responds when called.
Responds when called, but is often too willing to make decisions on his own without asking advice.
No problems – some difficulties with supervising consultants, but I have always found him to be accessible and well organised.
Often late for clinics.

Again, the comments in Box 13.3 highlight some good points, but there are also serious problems. Perhaps underlying difficulties account for these problems (*see* Chapter 17). Highlight exactly what you expect, in terms of accessibility and turning up on time, and the sanctions for not following these expectations. You may set ground rules, as follows:

➤ *Punctuality and accessibility are very important when working here.*
➤ Spell out what you expect.
   — *We start at 8 am with the first patient booked.*
   — *When you are the on-call doctor you are available and here in the building and contactable.*
   — *You need to be here by 7.50 am and ready to start for the 8 am appointment.*
➤ Monitor what actually happens.
➤ If your expectations are not met, spell out the sanctions.
➤ Measurement and feedback are the key strategies here.

Create and agree a plan with the learner. Explain the improvements required and the reasons underlying these. Highlight your standards, outline what you expect and write it all down. It is essential to check what is happening – to measure it and to feed it back to the learner.

TEACHING TEACHERS HOW TO GIVE CONSTRUCTIVE FEEDBACK

You can best learn how to give effective feedback through practice. Sometimes structured models feel artificial and unhelpful until you develop a language and series of phrases to help. It is also useful to seek and then reflect on feedback given to you by others, and to think about helpful aspects of what was said and the aspects that hindered you from improving your performance.

You could do this in several ways. Training courses that focus on developing feedback skills sometimes require participants to bring a practical skill to teach to another colleague, to give a five-minute lecture on a non-medical subject, or to appraise a trainee in a role-play situation using a prepared case scenario. In all of these settings, the teachers are watched by their colleagues and feedback is given at the end of the activity. It is especially useful for the person who is role-playing the trainee to give feedback. Sometimes colleagues launch straight into criticism of faults, and need to be reminded that they must state good points first, and only later discuss points which need to be improved, in a helpful and constructive way. One drawback of these exercises is that participants can get lost in the content and forget to talk about the process. Facilitators need to draw the discussion back to how the teaching was done, so that observers can hone their feedback skills.

An increased understanding of the importance of including feedback on people's strengths and how to give feedback constructively using one of the models available will improve the educational climate in your organisation. This can improve the learning outcomes, as well as the competence and motivation of your learners.

REFERENCES

1　Rowntree D. *Educational Technology in Curriculum Development*. 2nd edn. London: Paul Chapman Publishing; 1982.
2　Hore T. Teaching the teachers. *Anaesth Intensive Care*. 1976; **4**: 329–31.
3　Black P, William D. Assessment and classroom learning. *Assess Educ*. 1998; **5**: 7–73.
4　Parry KM. The doctor as teacher. *Med Educ*. 1987; **21**: 512–20.
5　Metcalfe DH, Matharu M. Students' perceptions of good and bad teaching: report of a critical incident study. *Med Educ*. 1995; **29**: 193–7.
6　Irby DM. Teaching and learning in ambulatory care settings – a thematic review of the literature. *Acad Med*. 1995; **70**: 898–931.
7　Rotem A, Godwin P, Du J. Learning in hospital settings. *Teach Learn Med*. 1995; **7**: 211–17.
8　Bedford H, Phillips T, Robinson J *et al*. *Assessment of Competencies in Nursing and Midwifery Education and Training*. London: English National Board for Nursing, Midwifery and Health Visiting; 1993.
9　Standing Committee on Postgraduate Medical and Dental Education. *Teaching Hospital Doctors and Dentists to Teach: its role in creating a better learning environment*. London: Standing Committee on Postgraduate Medical and Dental Education; 1992.
10　Lowry S. What's wrong with medical education in Britain? *BMJ*. 1992: **305**: 1277–80.
11　Lowry S. Teaching the teachers. *BMJ*. 1993; **306**: 127–30.
12　Coles C. Developing medical education. *Postgrad Med J*. 1993; **69**: 57–63.
13　Wall D, McAleer S. Teaching the consultant teachers – identifying the core content. *Med Educ*. 2000; **34**: 131–8.
14　Rolfe I, McPherson J. Formative assessment: how am I doing? *Lancet*. 1995; **345**: 37–9.
15　Stuart C. *Assessment, Supervision and Support in Clinical Practice: a guide for nurses, midwives and other health professionals*. Edinburgh: Churchill Livingstone; 2003.
16　Bailey J. The supervisor's story: from expert to novice. In: Johns C, Freshwater D, eds. *Transforming Nursing Through Reflective Practice*. London: Blackwell Science; 1998.
17　Pendleton D, Schofield T, Tate P *et al*. *The Consultation: an approach to teaching and learning*. Oxford: Oxford Medical Publications; 1984.
18　Standing Committee on Postgraduate Medical and Dental Education. *Appraising Doctors and Dentists in Training*. London: Standing Committee on Postgraduate Medical and Dental Education; 1996.
19　Brukner H, Altkorn DL, Cook S *et al*. Giving effective feedback to medical students: a workshop for faculty and house staff. *Med Teacher*. 1999; **21**: 161–5.
20　Wood L, Hassell A, Whitehouse A *et al*. A literature review of multi-source feedback systems within and without health services, leading to ten tips for their successful design. *Med Teacher*. 2006; **28**: e185–191.

21 Bullock AD, Hassell A, Markham WA *et al*. How ratings vary by staff group in multi-source feedback assessment of junior doctors. *Med Educ.* 2009; **43**: 516–20.

22 Whitehouse AB, Hassell A, Bullock A *et al*. 360 degree assessment (multisource feedback) of UK trainee doctors: field testing of team assessment of behaviours (TAB). *Med Teacher.* 2007; **29**: 171–6.

CHAPTER 14

Assessment

This chapter presents some of the issues in the area of assessment of learning:
➤ assessment – explanation of basic terms and principles
➤ domains of learning
➤ features of assessments.

The use of technology in assessment is discussed in Chapter 9.

ASSESSMENT
Explanation of the basic terms

'Assessment' is the term used to refer to the processes and instruments that are applied to measure the learner's achievements, normally after they have worked through a learning programme.

Assessment is a hurdle to be passed to allow progress to the next stage. This is 'pass' or 'fail', and is usually called 'summative' assessment, i.e. it 'sums up' achievement at the end of a period of study. This distinguishes it from formative assessment, which 'informs' you of achievements as you go along, highlighting progress and areas to develop while there is still time to do something about it (otherwise known as appraisal; *see* Chapter 15).

Assessment in the educational cycle

Remember the four simplified steps of the educational cycle:
1 Identify needs
2 Set objectives
3 Decide methods
4 Design assessment.

After you have identified learning needs, set your objectives and design your assessment tool(s) early on, so that both you and the learner are clear about what you are working towards. You will then have a way to test the learner at the end to establish whether they have succeeded or not – and the learner will also know what to expect.

Link between aims and objectives and assessment

The first step in designing an assessment tool is curriculum development (*see* Chapter 7). In everyday language, 'aims' and 'objectives' are synonymous – they are 'those things that we work towards.' However, in education we make a distinction between them. If you are setting aims and objectives for your learners, you need to know the specific meanings of the terms.

➤ **Aims** are broad statements of intent. For example, you might aim to produce a competent nurse or an effective healthcare teacher. Aims specify the broad direction in which you want your learner to go, but they do not specify how far they have to go, how they will get there, or how they will know when they are there.

➤ **Objectives** are outcome measures, and are specific statements addressed at aspects of the aim. They are usually written in terms of what the learner will be able to do at the end of the course of study. For example, 'At the end of this post the nurse will be able to apply a dressing using a sterile technique.'

Objectives usually specifically describe desirable outcomes, so we can see clearly what our assessment tool needs to be able to measure. They may be subdivided even further into highly specific steps in each of the activities to be learned.[1]

Writing objectives are crucial to the effectiveness of the teaching process, to help to focus your curriculum design as well as for assessing learners. Often people set out to teach without having a clear idea in mind of exactly what they are planning to achieve. They decide, for example, to hold 'a tutorial on diabetes.' Without clear objectives it is impossible to choose the most appropriate teaching method, to know what content can be omitted, to be sure whether the teaching has worked or to know how to evaluate it. From the learner's perspective, clear objectives, framed as learning outcomes, help them to decide whether a course of study is for them and will suit their learning needs, help plan their study, choose what aspects to go into in depth and how to prepare for assessments. A tutorial on diabetes might aim to inform the learner about the importance of good diabetic control, with objectives such as to 'know what pathological complications can occur.' Or you may aim to increase awareness of self-monitoring techniques available to patients, with one of the objectives being to 'be able to discuss the pros and cons of different testing kits.'

Therefore objectives are usually written in behavioural terms – that is, a statement of what the satisfactory learner will be able to do at the end of the period of study. These outcomes need to be as specific as we can make them. Phrases like to 'know the difference between different forms of x' are not as effective as to 'be able to classify x into the three categories, (a), (b) and (c).'

Certain words in objective setting are best avoided, such as 'to understand', as it is much harder to demonstrate understanding and, although clearly necessary and not impossible, to devise an assessment tool to measure understanding. If you set a behavioural task in the objective such as to be able to list (recall), categorise (differentiate) and rank (prioritise), you are still testing learners' understanding, but you are also guiding them as to how to demonstrate it and help you to assess it.

DOMAINS OF LEARNING

In one of the earliest attempts to produce a systematic classification of the types of learning, Bloom led a team of educationalists to devise 'Bloom's taxonomy.' He divided the three areas of learning into the cognitive domain (pertaining to intellectual processes), the 'psychomotor' domain (processes of physical skills) and the 'affective' domain (attitudinal and emotional processes).[2,3] More simply this may be thought of as:

➤ knowledge
➤ skills
➤ attitudes.

To be clear about what you are asking your learners to do, you need to consider which domain you are assessing and at which level – hence the importance of the wording of the objectives.

A taxonomy is a hierarchical and orderly classification in which each stage builds on the one above. For example, each domain, proceeding from the simple to the complex, can be subdivided (*see* Table 14.1). The affective domain proceeds from aspects outside the learner to more internal processes.

Focusing on Bloom's taxonomy of the cognitive domain, Table 14.2 provides illustrations of what skills might be demonstrated at each level of competence, and some of the appropriate words that you might incorporate into your objectives.[2] Once you have ordered these concepts, you can assign appropriate assessment tools.

The words in the objective column are used in the assessment process. They help you to define each competence:

➤ **Knowledge:** the remembering (recalling) of appropriate, previously learned information.
➤ **Comprehension:** grasping (understanding) the meaning of informational materials.
➤ **Application:** the use of previously learned information in new and concrete situations to solve problems that have single or best answers.
➤ **Analysis:** breaking down informational materials into their component parts, examining (and trying to understand the organisational structure of) such information to develop divergent conclusions by identifying motives or causes, making inferences and/or finding evidence to support generalisations.

TABLE 14.1 Subdivisions of the domains of learning

Level	Domain		
	Knowledge	**Skills**	**Attitudes**
Base level	Knowledge	Observation	Receiving (listening)
	Comprehension	Imitation	Responding
Application	Application	Practising	Valuing (advocating, defending)
Problem solving	Analysis	Mastering	Organisation
	Synthesis	Adapting	Characterisation (judging)
	Evaluation		

TABLE 14.2 The cognitive domain

Competence	Skills demonstrated	Objectives
Knowledge	Observation and recall of information Mastery of subject matter	List, define, tell, describe, identify, show, label, collect, examine, tabulate, quote, name, who, when, where, etc.
Comprehension	Understand information, grasp meaning, translate knowledge into new context, interpret facts, compare, contrast, order, group, infer causes, predict consequences	Summarise, describe, interpret, contrast, predict, associate, distinguish, estimate, differentiate, discuss, extent
Application	Use information, use methods, concepts and theories in new situations, solve problems using acquired skills or knowledge	Apply, demonstrate, calculate, complete, illustrate, show, solve, examine, modify, relate, change, classify, experiment, discover
Analysis	Seeing patterns, reorganisation of parts, recognition of hidden meanings, identification of components	Analyse, separate, order, explain, connect, classify, arrange, divide, compare, select, explain, infer
Synthesis	Use old ideas to create new ones, generalise from given facts, relate knowledge from several areas, predict, draw conclusions	Combine, integrate, modify, rearrange, substitute, plan, create, design, invent, 'what if?', compose, formulate, prepare, generalise, rewrite
Evaluation	Compare and discriminate between ideas, assess value of theories, presentations, make choices based on reasoned argument, verify value of evidence, recognise subjectivity	Assess, decide, rank, grade, test, measure, recommend, convince, select, judge, explain, discriminate, support, conclude, compare, summarise

➤ **Synthesis:** creatively or divergently applying prior knowledge and skills to produce a new or original whole.
➤ **Evaluation:** judging the value of material based on personal values/opinions, resulting in an end product with a given purpose, without real right or wrong answers.

CHOOSING ASSESSMENT TOOLS

Miller[4] has described four levels of assessment in healthcare (*see* Chapter 7):
➤ knows
➤ knows how
➤ shows how
➤ does.

Different assessments work better for different domains, and a common mistake is to mismatch domain and assessment tool. For example, assessment of practical resuscitation skills will be less successful if learners are asked to write an essay than if a mock scenario is arranged. Similarly, asking candidates at interview to give a lecture presentation on a specific topic is not the best way to assess communication skills with patients and colleagues.

The following sections show the match between some examples of assessment of competence within each domain of learning as applied to the healthcare setting.[5,6]

Knowledge

Information retention is best tested using a multiple-choice questionnaire (MCQ). Higher levels from comprehension to evaluation can be tested by means of extended matching questions, modified essay questions, scholarly essays, portfolio-based assessments and vivas. However, although vivas are commonly used in higher professional assessments, they are fraught with difficulties in terms of both reliability and validity.[7] Encouraging critical reflection and self-assessment might help learners to develop through these higher levels just as much as working towards a summative assessment.

Skills

The following tools all have a place in the assessment of learners' ability to demonstrate, show mastery of or adapt practical skills.

➤ **Consultation/communication skills:** standardised patients, objective structured clinical examination (OSCE; see below), teacher observation in daily work (video).
➤ **Presentation skills:** audience feedback.
➤ **Clinical procedures:** OSCE, teacher observation, and audit of case records, note-keeping, letters and summaries.
➤ **Use of investigations or data handling:** audit of case notes, OSCE, teacher observation in daily work.

Attitudes

Attitudes, beliefs and values are difficult, but not impossible, to assess. They need a performance rather than a competence assessment, which in turn requires us to define the ideal, the acceptable and the not acceptable, in relation to what we expect.

You may have experience of a learner who is polite and courteous to their trainer, but who is inconsiderate, rude, aggressive and overbearing to other trainees, healthcare staff and secretaries. Be aware of this, because it reflects a misunderstanding of being a member of a non-hierarchical healthcare team, and because it might have an impact on patient care.

Personal qualities, such as relationships with patients and colleagues, punctuality and courtesy, ethical values and belief systems, are all important attitudes for learners to acquire. Other difficult areas to assess include a learner's understanding of 'professionalism' and knowledge and application of medico-legal matters. Increasingly, these are being addressed in healthcare curricula, and ethics courses are becoming ever more popular. However, assessment processes lag behind. Knowing about something is not the same as believing it or carrying it out. To assess these attitudes you require information from those in a position to judge (e.g. patients, senior colleagues, peers and possibly multi-disciplinary colleagues). Bias can be minimised by ensuring that assessment is performed by more than one person where possible. Criteria, standards and tools need to be carefully developed to ensure that they are fit for purpose.

Assessments: desirable criteria

The ideal assessment is probably not achievable in real life, but certain principles can help to make assessments as fair as possible. The 'ideal' assessment should be:

➤ **valid:** it measures what it is supposed to measure (if it has face validity as well, it also appears to the learner as if it is measuring what it purports to measure)
➤ **reliable:** it measures it with essentially the same result each time (learners with the same level of performance will be judged equally regardless of who administers the assessment)
➤ **practicable:** it is easy to perform in terms of cost, time and skills of the assessors
➤ **fair to the learners and the teachers:** for example, differences between learners which are irrelevant to the subject that is being assessed do not affect the result, marking is not unnecessarily burdensome for teachers
➤ **useful to the learners and the teachers:** for example, it discriminates between good and poor candidates
➤ **acceptable:** in terms of, for example, cultural and gender issues
➤ **appropriate:** to what has been taught and learned on the programme.

The reliability and validity of assessments may increase when two trained assessors observe the same activity.[8]

Sometimes there is a trade-off between validity and reliability, an increase in one often occurring at the expense of the other. For example, consider MCQs for communication skills. They are very reliable, equally performing learners will score equally, but they will have low validity. The extent to which they can measure communication skills is low. At the other extreme you can increase validity by introducing simulated (or real) patients, but reliability will fall off, as you cannot ensure that learners of similar ability will score equally across all of the simulated patients.

This subject of psychometrics is well beyond the scope of this book. However, you should be aware that requests for reliability to be demonstrated in terms of statistical measurements are common.[9] For any assessment, there is true score and error. Classical test theory groups all of the errors together, and provides a measure of the levels of internal consistency (such as Cronbach's alpha). A value of 0.8 or above is regarded as acceptable for a high-stakes assessment. Generalisability theory has developed this concept further, and separates out the different sources of error (such as that of the candidates, the examiners and the different questions). Again, a generalisability coefficient of 0.8 or above is regarded as acceptable. In addition, generalisability theory can predict what the reliability would be if we increased or decreased the numbers of questions or examiners in an assessment. For example, a five-station OSCE with a low reliability of only 0.5 can be improved by increasing the number of stations to 20, which would improve the reliability to 0.8.

Norm referencing and criterion referencing

Whichever tool you use, you must decide how good is good enough. Norm-referenced tests rate a learner's performance alongside the performances of others at that stage in the same cohort – judgement is by comparison with each other. These tests give a less accurate representation of what each student can do, cannot provide useful feedback in terms of specific strengths and weaknesses, and are not an encouragement for group learning – rather they encourage competition.

An example may be a test that the top 25% pass, whatever their score. Sometimes an individual mark is compared with the group average to rank learners. Such tests are often used to control entry to the next stage of training, in order to limit numbers.

Criterion referencing rates learners' performances to determine whether they have achieved mastery. Very often it is done as a form of formative assessment, and it does not matter what their rank order is so long as they have achieved the competency. Clear behavioural objectives are required to define what the learner should know or be able to do, and standards of acceptable performance should be set.

OBJECTIVE STRUCTURED CLINICAL EXAMINATION (OSCE)

Since the late 1970s,[10] OSCEs have become a reliable way to assess basic clinical skills. In terms of Miller's pyramid (*see* Chapter 7), an OSCE assesses competence (*shows how*) but not what the health professional does in the workplace. It consists of a circuit of stations where candidates interact with materials, equipment or standardised patients (*see* Chapter 20). It can also be used as a practice opportunity. As a rough rule of thumb, 20 stations or 100 minutes of OSCE time may be needed to achieve an acceptable level of reliability.

The number of stations needs to be balanced. Too few stations will result in unreliable scores, whereas too many will give unmanageable numbers of marks and organisational headaches. Each station requires three components:
➤ the **stem** – this sets the scene for the learner and clearly states the task and the time available
➤ the **checklist** – for the assessor to score the performance, as detailed and specific as necessary to ensure reliability
➤ **background to the station** – e.g. instructions to simulated patients, model answers, information to be revealed in response to learners' observations.

Factors that affect reliability include the following:
➤ too few stations or too little testing time
➤ checklists or items that do not discriminate (too easy or too hard)
➤ inconsistent performance by simulated patients
➤ examiners who score idiosyncratically
➤ administrative problems (e.g. poor organisation, noise).

Factors that affect validity include the following:
➤ whether the problems are relevant and important; whether they are aligned with programme outcomes
➤ whether the stations will assess skills that have been taught
➤ whether content experts have reviewed the stations.

PORTFOLIOS[11]

Portfolios are personal collections of evidence from practice, demonstrating that a learner has met the learning outcomes or performance indicators (*see* Chapter 1). They are increasingly being used in clinical practice to demonstrate competence, and they work well as a formative assessment tool.

As summative assessment tools, portfolios generally have reasonably high levels of validity, because learners construct them to demonstrate particular learning outcomes that matter to them. They may be less reliable, due to their variation and the time taken to assess them. A specified structure and a clear assessment policy will help to make them fairer.

Criteria for assessment might include minimum and maximum word counts, time limits on items that are valid for inclusion, required items for inclusion or required numbers of types of material, and the presence and degree of reflective self-evaluative documentary evidence. Portfolios tend to be rated in terms of satisfactory completion or referral (requiring resubmission), as it is very difficult to make finer judgements about performance.

OBSERVATION OF PRACTICE[12]

When assessing the competent clinical practice of healthcare professionals, direct observation of real-life practice 'samples' performance and makes an inference about competence. This is based on the concept that competence is not directly observable, but can be inferred from successful behaviour. Assessors must position themselves to be able to accumulate enough evidence to make a judgement, since not all practice can be observed. The assessment may be of practical skills, behaviours and behaviour patterns, but these may also indicate the underlying attitudes and values held by the learner.

An ability to perform is only one aspect of competence, and questioning frequently complements observation to gain further, indirect evidence of competence that is 'hidden' and not available to observation.

Guidelines from the English National Board for Nursing, Midwifery and Health Visiting (published in 1997) state that the assessor should directly observe pre-registration nursing, midwifery and health visitor students for a minimum period of two days per working week, and pro rata for part-time workers.[13] Effective observation requires the assessor to:

➤ use a checklist
➤ allow enough time
➤ be aware of observer bias
➤ be aware of observer effect (observation will inevitably change practice)
➤ complement observation with other forms of assessment.

Advantages of observation
➤ Observation of practice can provide a high level of integrated assessments, testing several competences at the same time.
➤ It allows assessment of attitudes and interpersonal skills.
➤ It offers realistic evidence of competence.
➤ It allows assessment of problem-solving skills.

Disadvantages of observation
➤ The circumstances of observation may be too specific.
➤ It is lengthy and costly if reliability is to be assured.
➤ Only indirect evidence of knowledge and understanding is obtained.
➤ It does not assess ability to learn through practice and transfer skills to another setting.
➤ It is subject to observer bias and observer effect.

For some of these reasons, as well as others, such as the huge cost implications and lesser requirement for practical skills training, direct observation of actual practice does not occur widely in undergraduate training. Increasingly, however, postgraduate assessment processes include several observed competences and video recordings of consultations for external assessment – an extension of observation of practice.[14]

A review of postgraduate dental training[15] called for assessments utilising direct observation of clinical work to minimise criticism that the assessments are not well related to patient care. The other main findings were that attention needed to be given to aspects of:

➤ assessment that supports an integrated period of general professional training
➤ training and inspection of trainers, to minimise variation in assessment
➤ more 'authentic' assessments, to enhance the predictive value of the tests for future success.

WORKPLACE-BASED ASSESSMENTS

Workplace-based assessments measure what the healthcare professional does in day-to-day practice. In terms of Miller's pyramid (*see* Chapter 7), they measure *performance*. There has been a rapid increase in the use of such assessments in recent years. Such assessments include the mini-CEX, case-based discussion (CBD), direct observation of procedural skills (DOPS), procedure-based assessment (PBA), multi-source feedback (MSF, or 360° assessment), audit and patient satisfaction surveys.

Mini-clinical evaluation exercise (mini-CEX)

The mini-CEX assesses history taking, examination, communication skills, clinical judgement, professionalism, organisation and overall clinical care. A supervisor watches the learner carry out the patient interaction, and assesses them on a numerical scale. The mini-CEX is widely used in postgraduate medical training in the UK. However, there are problems with its reliability, as 12 to 14 ratings are needed to achieve a reliability of 0.8.[16] Difficulties also arise if there are no descriptors of what each of the points mean, and if there is no mention of which consultation model is to be used for history taking. Assessors need to be trained in the use of the tool and how to give feedback after each encounter.

Case-based discussion (CBD)[17]

Here the learner selects patient notes of cases that they have dealt with, and provides them for the trainer. The trainer then questions the learner on the case, and rates him or her in terms of medical record keeping, clinical assessment, investigation and referrals, treatment, follow-up and future planning, professionalism and overall clinical judgement. Again a numerical scale is used. As above, problems include a lack of descriptive anchors for the numerical scale, and problems with numbers needed for reliability.

Direct observation of procedural skills (DOPS)[17]

DOPS is designed for the assessment of clinical procedures (e.g. suturing) or investigations (e.g. lumbar puncture), and is widely used in postgraduate medical training. It has been designed to assess the learner's understanding of indications for the procedure/investigation, appropriate use of sedation or analgesia, technical ability, consideration for the patient, and management of complications. Again a numerical scale is used. When it has been tested, reliable results have been obtained with three observers each watching the learner undertaking two procedures. Variants of the tool have been produced, such as the Surgical DOPS, which is used for surgical and dental procedures.

Procedure-based assessment (PBA)[17]

For the assessment of more major surgical procedures, rather than using the DOPS (see above), the PBA is being used in surgical training.

> Really the only way to assess how good a surgeon is, is to come and watch him or her operate.

Within each of the surgical specialties a series of index operations has been developed. In orthopaedics, these may include carpal tunnel decompression, hip replacement, knee arthroscopy, etc. Assessed areas include obtaining informed consent, pre-operative planning, pre-operative preparation, exposure and closure, intra-operative technique and post-operative management. An experienced surgeon will observe the learner and provide appropriate supervision, assessment and feedback. Assessment is on a simple scale of *satisfactory* or *unsatisfactory and needing improvement*, or *not observed*. Information on reliability is not yet available.

CLINICAL AUDIT

Audit is a professional responsibility of UK doctors.[18] As discussed in Chapter 5, clinical audit is a process used to improve the quality of care through a series of steps including standard setting, measuring your performance, reviewing your work, implementing change and re-measuring your work after making these changes. Structured formats have been developed to guide the preparation and presentation of audits, and for the marking of audit projects.

Two simple and widely used audit assessment tools[18] that enable the marking of an audit project are described below. Reliability assessment found that 6 eight-criteria audits are necessary to give a generalisability coefficient of 0.8, and 14 such audits are necessary to yield a generalisability coefficient of 0.9. So one audit is not really enough!

The five-criteria audit schedule

Each of five criteria needs to be present to pass the assessment. The five criteria are as follows:

1 **reason for choice:** clearly defined, reflected in the title, and potential for change
2 **criteria chosen:** relevant to the subject of the audit and justifiable (e.g. on the basis of the literature)
3 **preparation and planning:** shows appropriate teamwork and methodology, and if standards are set they should be appropriate and justified
4 **interpretation of data:** uses relevant data to allow appropriate conclusions to be drawn
5 **detailed proposals for change:** shows explicit details of proposed changes.

This assessment does not require a complete audit cycle, so it can be used when learners are only in a post for a short time, and cannot re-examine practice after changes have been put in place.

The eight-criteria audit schedule

All eight criteria must be present for a pass to be awarded. The criteria are similar to the five criteria described above, but include a second data collection and conclusions about the lessons learned. The eight criteria are as follows:
1 **reasons for choice of audit:** potential for change and relevant to practice
2 **criteria chosen:** relevant to audit subject and justifiable (e.g. on basis of current literature)
3 **standards set:** targets towards a standard with a suitable timescale
4 **preparation and planning:** evidence of teamwork and adequate discussion where appropriate
5 **data collection 1:** results compared against the standard
6 **changes to be evaluated:** actual example described
7 **data collection 2:** comparison with data collection 1 and the standard
8 **conclusions:** summary of the main lessons learned.

PATIENT SATISFACTION SURVEYS

Patients may not be able to assess all aspects of a healthcare professional's performance, but they do prefer individuals with excellent communication skills and sound up-to-date technical skills. The patient satisfaction survey is increasingly viewed as a key component in measuring the quality of the performance of healthcare professionals. In UK general practice, patient satisfaction surveys (in the form of the General Practice Assessment Questionnaire (GPAQ); www.gpaq.info) are widely used, and are part of the assessment of general practitioner trainees (Patient Satisfaction Questionnaire (PSQ); www.rcgp.org.uk). Much larger numbers of assessments are needed to achieve reliability when compared with other workplace-based assessments. The GPAQ measures various aspects of care, including access to care, and not just the doctor–patient relationship. At least 50 completed GPAQs and 40 PSQs are required to obtain reliable results.

While completing the PSQ, patients are asked to rate the healthcare professional in 10 areas (plus a global assessment) using a seven-point scale (poor to fair, fair, fair to good, good, very good, excellent, and outstanding). The 10 areas are as follows:
1 making you feel at ease
2 letting you tell your story
3 really listening
4 being interested in you as a whole person
5 fully understanding your concerns
6 showing care and compassion
7 being positive
8 explaining things clearly
9 helping you to take control
10 making a plan of action with you.

MULTI-SOURCE FEEDBACK (MSF) (360° ASSESSMENT)

MSF is a very valid and reliable method of assessing attitudes and behaviours, and of detecting poor performance.[19] MSF collects evidence about the learner's communication skills with patients and with colleagues, teamworking, accessibility and professional behaviours. It is widely used in postgraduate medicine.[20] More detailed information on MSF can be found in Chapter 13.

ASSESSMENT AS AN EDUCATIONAL DEVICE

Assessment highlights to learners what is important. If you say that a subject will be assessed and make it a hurdle that needs to be passed in order to make progress, learners will study it, whether it is relevant or not! Learners work to pass the assessment that they know is coming.

You must set objectives that are aligned (i.e. help to build towards the overall aims of the course) and relevant (i.e. worth studying, and measurable). Identify the criteria that you will assess and the standards that will apply to those criteria, and devise effective tools to measure them.

Tips from experienced teachers

Some people use the terms 'assessment', 'appraisal' and 'evaluation' interchangeably, causing confusion about these activities. In part this arises from these words having similar meanings in everyday life. However, in education they each have explicit meanings, and you should ensure that your approach fits the intended purpose.

REFERENCES

1 Rowntree D. *Educational Technology in Curriculum Development.* 2nd edn. London: Paul Chapman Publishing; 1982.
2 Bloom BS. *Taxonomy of Educational Objectives. 1. Cognitive domain.* New York: David McKay; 1956.
3 Beard R, Hartley J. *Teaching and Learning in Higher Education.* London: Paul Chapman Publishing; 1984.
4 Miller GE. The assessment of clinical skills/competence/performance. *Acad Med.* 1990; **65:** s63–7.
5 Rolfe I, McPherson J. Formative assessment: how am I doing? *Lancet.* 1995; **345:** 837–9.
6 Black P, William D. Assessment and classroom learning. *Assess Educ.* 1998; **5:** 7–73.
7 Wakeford R. Principles of assessment. In: Fry H, Ketteridge S, Marshall S, eds. *Teaching and Learning in Higher Education.* London: Kogan Page; 1999.
8 Harden RM. Do you know? *Med Teacher.* 1999; **21:** 109.
9 Streiner DL, Norman GE. *Health Measurement Scales: a practical guide to their management and use.* 3rd edn. Oxford: Oxford University Press; 2003.
10 Harden RM, Gleeson FA. Assessment of clinical competence using an objective structured clinical examination (OSCE). *Med Educ.* 1979; **13:** 41–54.
11 Fry H, Ketteridge S, Marshall S. *Teaching and Learning in Higher Education.* London: Kogan Page; 1999.
12 Stoker D. Assessment in learning. (iii) Methods of assessment. *Nurs Times.* 1994; **90:** iii–viii.

13 English National Board for Nursing, Midwifery and Health Visiting. *Standards for the Approval of Higher Education Institutions and Programmes.* London: English National Board; 1997.

14 United Kingdom Conference of Postgraduate Advisers in General Practice. *Summative Assessment General Practice Training. The Blue Book.* London: Committee of General Practice Education Directors; 2003.

15 Morris Z, Bullock AD, Belfield C *et al.* Assessment in postgraduate dental education: an evaluation of strengths and weaknesses. *Med Educ.* 2001; **35**: 537–43.

16 Holmboe ES, Hawkins RE, Huot SJ. Effects of training in direct observation of medical residents' clinical competence: a randomized trial. *Ann Intern Med.* 2004; **140**: 874–81.

17 Davis MH, Ponnamperuma G, Wall D. Workplace-based assessment. In: Dent J, Harden RH, eds. *A Practical Guide for Medical Teachers.* 3rd edn. Oxford: Churchill Livingstone; 2009. pp. 341–55.

18 Lough JRM, Murray TS. Audit and summative assessment: a completed audit cycle. *Med Educ.* 2001; **35**: 363–75.

19 Wood L, Hassell A, Whitehouse A *et al.* A literature review of multi-source feedback systems within and without health services, leading to ten tips for their successful design. *Med Teacher.* 2006; **28**: e185–91.

20 Whitehouse AB, Hassell A, Bullock A *et al.* 360 degree assessment (multisource feedback) of UK trainee doctors: field testing of team assessment of behaviours (TAB). *Med Teacher.* 2007; **29**: 171–6.

FURTHER READING

* International Association for Medical Education. *ESME Assessment Course.* www.amee.org/index.asp?lm=95

* Jackson N, Jamieson A, Khan A. *Assessment in Medical Education and Training: a practical guide.* Oxford: Radcliffe Publishing; 2007.

* Quality Assurance Agency for Higher Education. *Code of Practice for the Assurance of Academic Quality and Standards in Higher Education. Section 6: Assessment of students.* 2nd edn. Mansfield: Quality Assurance Agency; 2006. www.qaa.ac.uk/academicinfrastructure/codeOfPractice/section6/COP_AOS.pdf

* Toolbox of Assessment Methods. www.acgme.org/Outcome/assess/Toolbox.pdf

CHAPTER 15

Appraisal

How am I doing? Appraisal meetings formalise this, by giving effective feedback (*see* Chapter 13) on a one-to-one basis between teacher and learner, in protected time set aside at regular intervals throughout the training programme. Appraisal builds on all of the supervision and feedback skills covered in earlier chapters, but is certainly not a substitute for close supervision and feedback on day-to-day work.

Appraisal (sometimes, confusingly, called formative assessment by educationalists) has been defined as a two-way dialogue focusing on the personal, professional and educational needs of the parties, which produces agreed outcomes.[1] It is a process of regular reviews between teacher and learner, with support, carried out for the learner's benefit. Appraisal, through reflecting on practice, allows both the demonstration of strengths and the revealing of difficulties, so that the former may be reinforced and the latter can be put right within the framework of the objectives that were set at the start of the programme. Appraisal is non-threatening, friendly and supportive, and does not result in a judgement or a pass/fail decision. It is sometimes called facilitated self-appraisal.

This chapter covers the concepts involved in appraisal of a learner and, more specifically, a learner who is junior to you. However, you can use the information to prepare for your own appraisals and appraisals of peers.

BACKGROUND TO APPRAISAL

Formative assessment has been extensively used for healthcare professionals in training. It helps to identify what learners have achieved, might achieve and are now ready to achieve.[2] Learners are actively involved in reflecting on their practice, discussing it and sharing ideas about how to develop further towards learning goals. There is a degree of mutuality about the process (sometimes called 'feed-forward'), where teachers collect information and insights into the educational opportunities that they provide.

Appraisal is relevant to and undertaken by healthcare professionals across different disciplines and countries. Appraisal is now a contractual requirement for all UK doctors to maintain their personal and professional development. Peer appraisal differs slightly from formative assessment, mainly in the nature of the relationship between appraiser and appraisee and the degree to which the appraiser is responsible for the overall progress of the appraisee.

Appraisal for healthcare professionals differs from that in industry, as in the latter setting it is often used as a performance management tool, and is an uncomfortable mixture of development and judgement.

Appraisals are often undertaken by line managers, tutors, educational supervisors, preceptors or colleagues or peers who have been appointed and trained as appraisers,[3] depending upon the discipline in which the appraisee works and the seniority of the appraisee.

CHARACTERISTICS OF APPRAISAL

Table 15.1 lists the general principles of appraisal and shows how it compares with assessment, with which it is often confused.

TABLE 15.1 General principles of appraisal and assessment

Feature	Appraisal	Assessment
Prime purpose	Developmental 'Informing progress'	Judging achievement 'Summing up'
Participants	Appraiser and appraisee	Learner and third party
Methods used	Structured conversation	Varied (see Chapter 14)
Areas covered	Educational, personal and professional development, career progress, employment (appraisee's agenda)	Learning objectives (third-party agenda)
Process informed by	Appraisee's self-assessment, day-to-day observation by teachers, other work-related inputs, results of assessments and examinations	Outcome of standard, objective tests
Standards of achievement	Internal (personal to the appraisee) and negotiated with the appraiser	Pre-determined by assessing body
Output of the process	Record of appraisal having taken place, agreed educational and personal development plan	Pass/fail
Confidential to learner?	Yes, in most circumstances	No
Review/appeal	No need, as decisions should always be joint ones	Yes
Outcome	Enhanced education, personal and professional development	Proceed to next stage

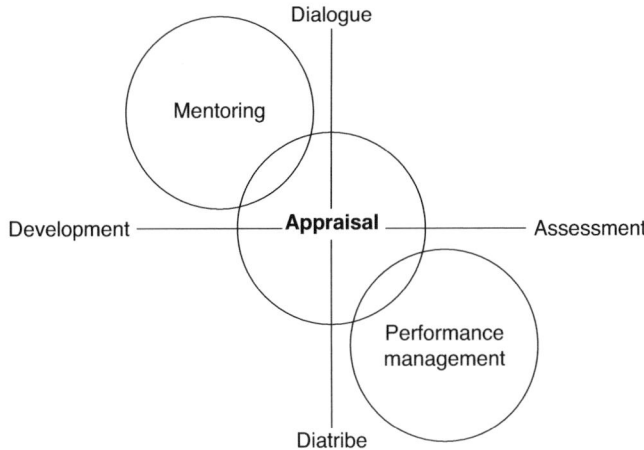

FIGURE 15.1

Questions to ask

Assessors should help the learner to understand their progress by asking the following questions.[4]

➤ Am I achieving statutory competences?
➤ Is there a demonstration of a growing level of skills?
➤ Is my performance consistent?
➤ Do I show a growing understanding of the principles underpinning practice?
➤ Am I demonstrating the development of attitudes and values appropriate to professional practice?
➤ Is there a demonstration of the ability to engage in reflective practice?

Any feedback on performance must consider the circumstances under which the learner is performing.[5]

The appraisal process has links with performance review, as it covers areas of statutory competence and progress, but it is also contextualised to the individual's professional circumstances and needs, and so has some features that overlap with mentoring (*see* Figure 15.1).[6]

CARRYING OUT APPRAISAL

A good working definition of appraisal is the provision of a structured process by which the learner can be helped to define their own learning needs in the light of information they can gather or be given about progress from whatever source. Plans can then be made to meet those needs.

Aims for the appraisal process with learners are as follows:
➤ To meet regularly. In the best schemes, progress is reviewed frequently (some specify every 2, 3, 4 or 6 months). Annual reviews are insufficient.
➤ To prevent information coming as a shock during a formal appraisal interview. Ongoing feedback will avoid this.
➤ To continue day-to-day supervision, support and feedback on performance.

➤ To ensure that the appraisee can achieve the agreed objectives and, where necessary, give or direct them to help.

➤ To set the learner's objectives within the overall framework of what staff in that grade are expected to achieve, or what learners at that stage are expected to be able to demonstrate.

➤ To curb the tendencies of unreasonably self-critical appraisees.

➤ On the whole, appraisal interviews are best conducted on a one-to-one basis.

➤ To respect any promised level of confidentiality. The only exception is where aspects of poor performance come to light when the appraiser has a professional responsibility to protect patients. This proviso should be made explicit at the start of the process.

The skills for successful appraisal

➤ Listen.

➤ Reflect back what is being said by the appraisee.

➤ Support.

➤ Counsel.

➤ Treat information in confidence.

➤ Inform without censuring.

➤ Judge constructively.

➤ Identify educational needs.

➤ Construct and negotiate achievable plans.

Listening is key. Remember what *listening* really means – keep your mouth closed and your ears and brain open, not interrupting, not dominating the conversation, and not going in with pre-judged ideas and conclusions already reached. The balance of talking in an appraisal interview should be roughly 80:20 between the appraisee and the appraiser.

The appraisal discussion

Arrange a time when you are both free, and find a quiet room from which your conversation cannot be overheard. Appraisal needs to be prepared ahead and at least an hour set aside.

1 Collect information from:
   — the learner
   — the learner's log book
   — examination results
   — courses attended
   — publications and presentations
   — other teachers
   — other staff, both clinical and administrative.

2 Some prompts to reflect on for peer appraisal might include:
   — review of significant event analysis
   — review of audits and protocol development
   — review of prescribing data, referral data
   — working relationships with colleagues
   — any feedback from, or involvement of, patients

— review of teaching management and research activity
— last year's personal development plan and log of completed learning.
3 Agree on an agenda.
4 Structure the discussion using three domains. You might choose:
— knowledge
— skills
— attitudes.
5 Alternatively, use the competences identified in the core curriculum for their specialty or discipline.
6 Agree the current position. Reinforce strengths and identify problems.
7 Identify ways of resolving problems and other needs.
8 Agree a plan for the future.
9 Agree the date and time of the next appraisal meeting.

USING APPRAISAL TO DEAL WITH PROBLEMS

Sometimes problems concerning a learner are brought to you by others. The learner may not realise that there is a problem, and when told about it they may react angrily, deny the problem or accuse those making the comments of bias. This section provides advice on techniques to assist you in such circumstances. However, some learners lack insight to such an extent that you may require others to help you (*see* Chapter 17).

Even with peer appraisal you may sometimes need to address difficult areas, and may find it tricky to tackle these. As an appraiser, you have to make a decision. Are patients at risk? Does the appraisee lack insight? If the answer to both questions is yes, you must stop the appraisal and start your local poor performance procedure. If patients are not at direct risk and/or the colleague has insight and is prepared to stop working in that area while seeking some retraining, it may be possible to work on and make note of these issues. If the appraisee becomes angry or defensive, the appraisal should be stopped and referred to the appropriate risk management or clinical governance lead. In peer appraisal there is no obligation, as there would be in an educational supervisory position, to deal with it any further, except for your professional responsibilities in the case of a threat to patient safety.

Tips for dealing with problems with appraisal

1 **The whole process must be conducted using description, not judgement.** For example: *Description*: 'You have not attended 50% of the training sessions, and there have been three occasions when you were half an hour late for the start of the clinic.' *Judgement*: 'You seem to be lazy and disorganised.'
2 **A key point:** keep it friendly. Being descriptive allows you to assume the role of a concerned friend and adviser rather than an outraged boss. Your role is to nurture the learner and not necessarily to like them. Therefore ignore any verbal or non-verbal anger or aggression that you may feel. Show respect for the learner and it is more likely to be reciprocated.
3 **Identify and reinforce strengths.**
4 **Problem areas need exact definition, not generalisations.** For example: *Definition*: 'Your operations tend to take about 50% longer on average, and your knot tying in the cases I helped you with was insecure and different each time.'

Generalisation: 'You've got two left hands.'

Express the problem so as to obtain mutual agreement about how to proceed.

5 **Such agreement will be much enhanced by objective evidence.** For example, this might include witnessing of practical skills, team observation, written tests, case-note review or video.

6 **Collaborate on constructive solutions.** Each specific problem area should have an agreed method of targeted training, the setting of objectives to be achieved and a specified timescale.

7 **Identify 'carrots' and 'sticks' to promote achievement of objectives.** These must be realistic. If something you promise to aid achievement is not delivered, this will seriously demotivate the learner. If threatened sanctions are not applied, future threats will be less effective.

8 **Troubleshoot subsequent progress.** For instance, remove minor obstacles before they become major. Keep tabs on the situation – hoping of course to catch the learner doing things right! By taking these actions, when the time comes for review, everyone will be well aware of the expected outcome, and any necessary sanctions can be applied with less confrontation. Review regularly until the learner is back on course.

9 **Be unyielding in your minimum expectations.** If you have insisted that the trainee should attend 70% of a training programme and they do not comply, you must keep to the prearranged sanction.

Tips from experienced teachers

- Use description, not judgement.
- Keep it friendly, both verbally and non-verbally, even if you do not like the person.
- Identify and reinforce strengths.
- Precisely define and mutually agree on problems.
- Collect objective evidence.
- Collaborate on constructive solutions.
- Identify and use 'carrots' and 'sticks' to make it happen.
- Keep checking – preferably to catch the learner doing things right.
- Do not capitulate on your bottom line.

REFERENCES

1 Standing Committee on Postgraduate Medical and Dental Education. *Appraising Doctors and Dentists in Training.* London: SCOPME; 1996.

2 Torrance H, Pryor J. *Investigating Formative Assessment.* Buckingham: Open University Press; 1998.

3 Chambers R, Tavabie A, Mohanna K *et al. The Good Appraisal Toolkit for Primary Care.* Oxford: Radcliffe Publishing; 2004.

4 Stuart C. *Assessment, Supervision and Support in Clinical Practice: a guide for nurses, midwives and other health professionals.* Edinburgh: Churchill Livingstone; 2003.

5 Phillips T, Schostak J, Tyler J. *Practice and Assessment in Nursing and Midwifery: doing it for real.* London: English National Board for Nursing, Midwifery and Health Visiting; 2000.

6 Robinson P, Simpson L. *e-Appraisal: a guide for primary care*. Oxford: Radcliffe Medical Press; 2003.

FURTHER READING

* Chambers R, Tavabie A, Mohanna K *et al*. Being an effective appraiser. In: *The Good Appraisal Toolkit for Primary Care*. Oxford: Radcliffe Publishing; 2004.

CHAPTER 16

Evaluation

➤ Does the teaching programme achieve its objectives?
➤ What did the trainees think of the half-day release course?
➤ How are the junior posts performing in terms of training?
➤ How effective was the practical skills course you ran last month?

These are all evaluation questions. This chapter looks at what evaluation is and how it can be effectively performed.

Educational evaluation is a systematic approach to collection, analysis and interpretation of information about any aspect of conceptualisation, design, implementation and utility of educational programmes. Evaluation measures the teaching. It is not the same as measuring learning – that is assessment. However, the results of assessment processes can be incorporated into evaluation, and are particularly useful when trying to evaluate some of the higher-order outcomes, such as how your teaching transferred into the clinical practice of participants or impacted on healthcare.

Evaluation can focus on the effectiveness of a completed programme, when it is sometimes called product or summative evaluation and is often carried out by independent observers. Alternatively, we can look at programme quality, usually during the earlier stages, and this is sometimes called process or formative evaluation. This is often carried out by development personnel within the department.

Elements of evaluation can be undertaken by:
➤ learners[1]
➤ teachers
➤ a third party.

THE EVALUATION CYCLE[2]

Evaluation is a vital component of the educational process. Like any monitoring process, it is iterative. Without it, curricula cannot evolve and develop in response to changing needs, resource allocation cannot be decided, and professional development of teachers is more difficult. When applied to courses and study days, evaluation often aims to find out 'how the teacher did.' When applied to programmes, evaluation is often used to establish whether 'you are doing what you set out to do.'

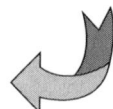

Teaching or learning activity planned
with evaluation in mind

Planning and preparation
to implement action

Collection and assessment
of evaluation data

Reflection and analysis,
agree on changes

FIGURE 16.1

Figure 16.1 shows the evaluation cycle. Reflect for a moment on your practice. Consider the feedback that you gather from your learners. At what stage are they asked for their comments? Does this give you time to respond to the issues that they raise? Can their comments affect your teaching or only the experience of those to follow? How often do you make changes in response to their comments? Do you receive useful information that helps you to make changes to the course design or your personal development? What sort of questions are you asking?

What about the courses or educational programmes that you run? How do you know whether you are meeting your aims overall? What happens to those who complete your courses? Are they performing better in the workplace? What could you do to increase the effectiveness of the learning experience?

Increasingly, learners and others are going to demand evidence that your teaching is robust and has been evaluated for performance.

When evaluating your teaching interventions, one of the difficulties is defining from which perspective you should look at outcomes. Evaluation has been grouped into student-oriented, programme-oriented, institution-oriented, programme-oriented

TABLE 16.1 Evaluating educational activities: the four levels[2]

Level	Evaluation of	Measure	Participant
1	Reaction	Satisfaction or happiness	What is the participant's response to the programme? What was the uptake of the course like? How many attended? Did they all complete the course?
2	Learning	Knowledge or skills acquired Modification of attitudes or perceptions	What did the participant learn?
3	Behaviour	Transfer of learning to workplace	Did the participant's learning affect their behaviour?
4	Results	Transfer or impact on society	Did changes in the participant's behaviour affect their organisation? Were there any benefits or problems noted as a result of these changes?

and stakeholder-oriented outcomes.[1] It is useful to think about your effectiveness in terms of the needs of these groups.

Kirkpatrick described a hierarchy of evaluation, or four levels on which to focus our questions (*see* Table 16.1),[3] and these have recently been adapted for use in healthcare education.[4]

PARTICIPANT EVALUATION

The quickest and most common form of evaluation is to ask for participant feedback. Evaluation forms given out at the end of a study day 'to help the organisers as they prepare for the next study day' are commonplace. Such forms usually include the following questions:
➤ Did today meet your expectations?
➤ What aspects went well or did not go well?
➤ What helped learning to occur or got in the way of learning?

We can now see that these are level 1 evaluative questions in the Kirkpatrick hierarchy. Sometimes the form will continue along the following lines:
➤ What three things did you learn on this course?
➤ What do you know now that you didn't know before?

These are level 2 questions. It is uncommon to be asked level 3 or 4 questions, such as 'What things have you changed at work as a result of this course?' and 'What has been the impact of changes that you have made?' Clearly, this is because these are delayed outcomes that cannot be evaluated on the day.

What topics might you ask the learner to evaluate?

Evaluative questions for participants can also be designed around the stages of the educational cycle.

Needs assessment
➤ Was the course relevant to you? Were needs met, or what was the extent of needs that were not met?
➤ Were problems solved, or what was the extent of problems still remaining? Or were problems not tackled?

Objectives setting
➤ Were the objectives clear?
➤ What important things were learned?
➤ What else did you need to know about?

Methods
➤ Were the methods appropriate (e.g. lectures, group work, presentations, practical sessions, etc.)?
➤ Obtain the learners' views of the lecturers and group facilitators. Could you read the slides during presentations? Was there time for discussions and asking questions? How good were the handouts?

Assessment

➤ What three things have you learned today?

➤ What was the take-home message?

Sadly, the opportunity for further development following learner evaluation is some-times limited by questions (or responses) at the level of other issues, such as food, timetables, communications, sound, documentation, ambience and car parking. The quality of the feedback may reflect the level of insight that the learners have into what a good educational experience would look or feel like for them, the degree to which they are confident about making judgements about their teachers, or some misunder-standing about the purpose of the questioning and how it will affect them. Sometimes, however, it is more to do with the quality of the questions and the level at which they are pitched.

Sometimes the best suggestions arise in free text comments. However, you must pose a stem question that is sufficiently inspiring to raise the level of the feedback. Consider asking 'What suggestions do you have to help this course really make an impact on patient care?' These are often things you had not thought about or included as struc-tured questions, and sometimes you will get real gems (or daft comments)!

Consider the evaluation form in Box 16.1. To what extent is it a good example of a form that will produce meaningful information that can aid development of the course?

BOX 16.1 Example of an evaluation form

Your thoughts and reflections on this day will provide valuable feedback for us as we look towards the next stage.

Satisfaction
- Did the day meet your expectations?
- What went well for you today?
- What could have gone better?

Knowledge and skills
- What do you know now that you didn't know before?
- What helped this learning to occur?
- What got in the way of learning?

Transfer of skills
- What will you do differently in your teaching/practice?

Impact
- How will your students/patients be affected by what you have learned on the course?

You don't have to evaluate everything

Sometimes evaluation forms attempt to evaluate every single thing in a course, using a very long and detailed questionnaire with complex marking scales. This is rarely nec-essary. Focus on things you can change. If you use the same form repeatedly, consider the type and amount of useful information that you are obtaining and whether the questions need to be pruned or altered.

Characteristics of a good evaluation question

A good evaluation question is:
➤ appropriate – relevant to the educational programme
➤ intelligible – can be understood clearly
➤ unambiguous – means the same thing to everyone
➤ unbiased – does not trigger one response selectively
➤ simple – contains only one idea per question
➤ ethical
➤ pitched at higher levels on the Kirkpatrick hierarchy.

An evaluation should be valid, reliable, simple, practical and probably anonymous. It can be either *quantitative* (numbers) or *qualitative* (descriptive), or both.[5,6]

Rating scales (e.g. Likert scales, semantic differential scales)

The Likert scale is a popular scale used by sociologists and psychologists in research. It consists of an opinion statement and is then followed by (usually) a five-point scale asking the respondent to indicate the extent to which they agree or disagree with that opinion statement. For example:

Please circle one of the numbers that best represents your view:					
I now feel much more confident in diagnosing asthma	1	2	3	4	5
(where 1 = strongly disagree, 5 = strongly agree)					

The semantic differential scale is somewhat different. A statement is given and the respondent is asked to rate it, usually on a seven-point scale, with adjectives such as *good–bad* at either end of the scale. For example:

Please circle one of the numbers that best represents your view:							
This course was pitched at just the right level for my needs	1	2	3	4	5	6	7
(where 1 = bad, 7 = good)							

Snowball review

A snowball review is a group-based evaluation method that takes participants through a number of formal steps during which their opinions and comments are elicited, shared, reviewed and compiled into a final list of strengths and weaknesses of the course. To begin with the participants work alone, reflecting for a few minutes about their experiences of the course. Each person should list three good points and three suggestions for improvement.

The participants should next form pairs and open discussions to reach a composite list of good points and suggestions for improvement. These lists could increase to four good and four bad points to accommodate divergent views.

Neighbouring pairs should merge to form units of four and talk their way to a new composite list. Groups of four should then merge to form groups of eight, or nearly eight, to tackle the task of arriving at another list of composite views. Then one member from each group of eight should report their agreed conclusions to the whole group. Alternatively, you can collect in one completed sheet from each group of eight, and later collate the results and feed them back to course members.

The strength of the snowball method is that it involves participants in contributing and discussing their views of the course. It also provides opportunities for them to feed these back to the course organiser or leader and to discuss them. A further strength is that it is tailored to the precise educational event in question. The weakness (and strength) of this method is that it is time-consuming, which means that it is largely inappropriate for short courses.

It can be used with groups of any size, but is particularly suitable as a way of ensuring the personal participation and contribution of all members of larger groups.

PEER REVIEW

Evaluation conducted by others who are not involved as learners in the teaching process is an important way to make revisions and modifications to your programme, and enables you to:
➤ determine effectiveness
➤ increase accountability
➤ assist in decision making.

You might ask such an individual to evaluate:
➤ you as course leader/instructor
➤ the whole programme, the form of instruction, or the technology
➤ the environment
➤ support services
➤ levels of use
➤ cost
➤ outcomes
➤ management
➤ curriculum materials
➤ the impact on learners.

Teaching evaluation

Peer review of the teaching process itself, having a colleague sit in and observe you as you teach, is a cornerstone of quality control in teaching institutions. As a method of personal and professional development for teachers, it is a powerful tool and is useful for evaluating the effectiveness of a course or even a department.

However, deciding how to measure the teaching under observation, and how to make judgements about efficacy, are not easy tasks. You need to consider what makes teaching effective (what criteria matter), how you will discriminate between good and excellent practitioners (what standards should be applied), and how can you spot effective teaching happening (decide what tools are needed).

Consider asking a colleague to observe and comment on your next teaching session.

Box 16.2 contains an evaluation document used in the peer and expert review components of the Postgraduate Certificate in Medical Education at Staffordshire University, which was adapted from the Higher Education Funding Council for England (HEFCE) monitoring forms.

BOX 16.2 Guidelines for review of a teaching session and collection of evidence, adapted from the HEFCE Guidance for Assessors

Before observing the session, discuss its purpose and structure with the teacher who is being assessed.

During observation, make notes relevant to the prompts given below. Do not expect them all to be relevant in every setting. At the end of the session ensure that feedback is given to the teacher.

Prompts:
1 What were the objectives of the session? Were they appropriate?
2 Did the teacher outline the structure and purpose of the session?
3 Did the teacher address the issue of the learners' needs?
4 Could the teacher be seen and heard?
5 Were the key points emphasised?
6 Were the explanations clear to the students?
7 Were the examples and analogies appropriate?
8 Was appropriate use made of audiovisual aids?
9 Was the session stimulating for the students?
10 Was there a variety of activities?
11 Did the teacher ask or invite questions or other forms of student participation?
12 Did the teacher cite references and/or refer to relevant research or scholarship?
13 Did the teacher summarise key points and conclusions?
14 Was the type of educational activity chosen appropriate to the learning outcomes?

Which of the following statements best summarises the class?
a) The session failed to make an acceptable contribution to the attainment of the learning objectives set.
b) The session made an acceptable contribution to the attainment of the learning objectives, but significant improvement could be made.
c) The session made a substantial contribution to the attainment of the learning objectives, but there is scope for improvement.
d) The session made a full contribution to the attainment of the learning objectives.

Report for review of a teaching session

Teacher:
. . . .

Observer:
. . . .

Teaching session reviewed:

. . . .

Date:

. . . .

1 Has the clinical teacher identified the specific learning objectives for this session (knowledge and understanding, key skills, cognitive skills, subject-specific, practical or professional skills)? What are they?
2 Comment on the strengths and weaknesses in relation to the learning objectives.

Prompts	Strengths	Weaknesses
Clarity of objectives		
Planning and organisation		
Methods/approach		
Delivery and pace		
Content (currency, accuracy, relevance, use of examples, level, match with students' needs)		
Student participation		
Use of accommodation and learning resources		

3 Summarise the overall quality of the session in relation to the learning objectives.

EXTERNAL EVALUATORS

Third-party review is the third type of evaluation.[7]

Objectives approach

This method looks for consistency or 'alignment' between goals, experiences and outcomes using a pre-test, post-test design. Behaviours can be measured by either norm-referenced or criterion-referenced tests. This approach measures the learner's progress against course aims.

The context, input, process and product (CIPP) approach

Information is collected from a variety of sources to provide a basis for making better decisions. This approach consists of the following four phases, which look at different aspects of an educational programme:

1 context
2 input
3 process
4 product.

Naturalistic evaluation

This model takes into account participants' definitions of key concerns and issues. Data collection is qualitative. It allows the learners to set the investigative agenda and determine the criteria for evaluation. Throughout, the language that is used and mode of presenting the findings are intended to be accessible to participants.

The timing of the evaluation of educational activities in relation to the timing of the activity is important. Self-reported satisfaction with courses fades over time, as participants return to work and find it hard to implement changes that they may have learned on the course. Therefore good outcome scores in early evaluation may not be sustained, or achieved, if evaluation is carried out too long after the event. Similarly, later, less good performance in evaluation may give a better overall judgement about the impact of the course. So deciding which aspects to measure, and which marker to use and when, are integral to the success of an evaluation tool.

Tips from experienced teachers

Get used to the idea of critiquing your teaching by videoing yourself and carrying out a self-evaluation first. It is an effective way of demonstrating your commitment to professional development in your personal development plan.

REFERENCES

1 General Medical Council. *Tomorrow's Doctors*. London: General Medical Council; 2009.
2 Wilkes M, Bligh J. Evaluating educational interventions. *BMJ*. 1999: **318**: 1269–72.
3 Kirkpatrick DI. Evaluation of training. In: Craig R, Mittel I, eds. *Training and Development Handbook*. New York: McGraw Hill; 1967.
4 Barr H, Freeth D, Hammick M. *Evaluations of Interprofessional Education: a United Kingdom review of health and social care*. London: United Kingdom Centre for the Advancement of Interprofessional Education with the British Educational Research Association; 2000.
5 Bowling A. *Research Methods in Health: investigating health and health services*. Buckingham: Open University Press; 1997.
6 Bramley P. *Evaluating Training*. London: Institute of Personnel and Development; 1996.
7 Grant J, Frances S. *The Effectiveness of Continuing Professional Development*. London: Joint Centre for Education in Medicine; 1999.

FURTHER READING

• Best Evidence Medical Education (BEME). Report of meeting, 3–5 December 1999, London. *Med Teacher*. 2000; **22**: 242–5.

CHAPTER 17

The challenging trainee

THE DIFFICULT STUDENT, DOCTOR, NURSE OR THERAPIST: HOW TO ADDRESS THE PROBLEM

Sometimes it all goes wrong. What should you do when you think you have tried everything and are still struggling with a learner who is not learning or performing well, or who is disrupting group learning? Other teachers can help by sharing the problem with you. Don't keep the problem to yourself, and don't postpone addressing it until the end of the learner's time with you. This chapter offers a way to approach such challenges, which might help to tease out and remedy the problems.

Sometimes the difficulty lies with the learner, sometimes with the teacher and sometimes with the learner–teacher relationship. There are probably as many causes of this as there are challenging trainees, but there are some recurring themes:

➤ mismatch between teaching style and stage of self-directedness of the learner
➤ mismatch of learning style between learner and teacher
➤ problems with the learning-group dynamics
➤ health-related issues (both physical and mental)
➤ learner and/or teacher's stressed state
➤ problems outside work (e.g. family difficulties, illness)
➤ disciplinary matters.

Multi-disciplinary healthcare teachers on a Postgraduate Certificate in Medical Education were asked what they found challenging about teaching. Some of their responses are listed in Box 17.1. You will probably recognise things that are true for you.

BOX 17.1 Challenges encountered when teaching

- Learners say 'yes' but mean 'no' when I ask whether they understand.
- People sit at the back of the group and talk throughout the session.
- Students relate to me on a surface level and don't incorporate learning into the next scenario.
- Juniors can't get on with other members of the team.
- Students forget what we have covered.

- I have a trainee who is competent clinically, but lazy.
- I have to give advice about moving/changing career.
- Learners know more than me!
- I need to find out what the trainee doesn't know.
- Learners react in an irritated manner or it turns into an argument.
- We can identify the issue but the learner doesn't want to address it.
- People don't listen to reason.
- I need to balance pastoral care/careers counselling with teaching and clinical commitments.
- Trainees say 'teach me something.'
- A trainee is not able to recognise weaknesses or shortcomings.
- I find it difficult to confront trainees with attitude problems.

One of the keys to preventing or dealing with difficulties lies in the educational rapport between the learner and the teacher. The Johari window (*see* Figure 17.1) is a model for thinking about communication.[1] (It also helps you to think about identification of learning needs; *see* Chapter 13.)

The four panes of the window represent how relationships are built up by an accumulation of information from 'self' and 'others' – me and you. As you build relationships with your learners to increase the effectiveness of your teaching, this model might help to explain why some people are considered to have communication difficulties, or are labelled poor communicators, or worse still, why relationships become dysfunctional. Up to a point, the larger the area called the arena in the top left-hand 'pane' of the window, the more productive the relationship will be.

Behaviour

Consider the crossed lines that separate the panes in the window in Figure 17.1 as if they can be moved in the direction of the arrows to vary pane size. The horizontal line represents exposure (disclosure). Here you open up the self, share ideas and

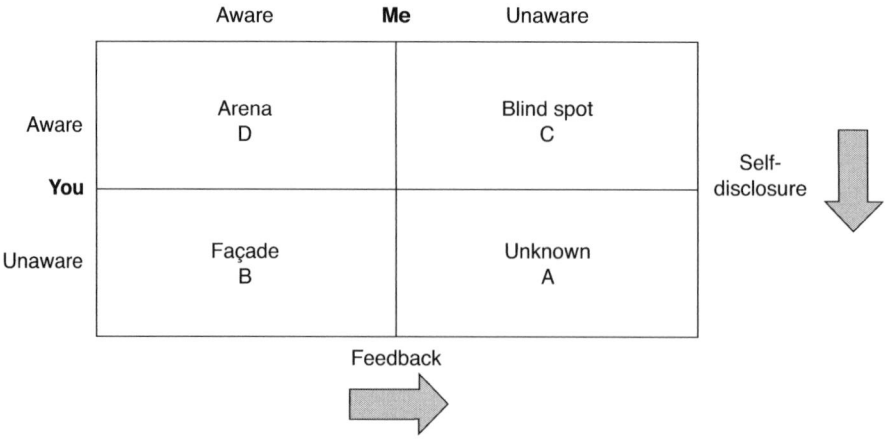

FIGURE 17.1

information, admit mistakes, and talk about feelings and opinions. As you increase exposure, your façade decreases, but the blind spot may increase due to less time being given to feedback.

The vertical line in Figure 17.1 represents feedback seeking. Here you ask for and encourage feedback, and the self gives others the opportunity to express their feelings in an open and supportive way. If used alone it may increase the façade, as it allows less time for exposure.

You can use either of these behaviours equally, but most people have a preference for one or the other. To enhance relationships you need not change, but alter the balance of these two basic behaviours.

➤ **Type A**: little exposure, little feedback seeking. These individuals are often perceived as withdrawn, aloof or impersonal, where the unknown square (in Figure 17.1) is the largest. This may induce resentment in others, who may take the behaviour personally. It is common in large bureaucratic organisations.

➤ **Type B**: increased feedback seeking, little exposure. These individuals decrease the information about themselves that is available to others, while requiring more from others, due to either fear or a wish for power or control. Others may react by withdrawing trust or becoming hostile.

➤ **Type C**: increased exposure, neglect of feedback. These individuals are oblivious to the effect that they have on others. They have a large blind spot, as the opportunity for feedback is rare. They may be confident of their own opinions, and insensitive, with little concern for the feelings of others. Listeners may become angry and reluctant to tell them anything.

➤ **Type D**: balanced. These individuals have a large arena, as feedback seeking and exposure are well used. They are open and candid. Initially others may be put on the defensive, but when they are seen as genuine, productive relationships can follow. They induce an open, balanced response in others.

Teachers and learners need to be sensitive about the covert content of the blind spot, the façade and the hidden area, and respect privacy concerning information that is kept hidden for reasons of social training or custom.

WHY HEALTH PROFESSIONALS RUN INTO DIFFICULTIES WITHIN THE EDUCATIONAL SETTING

Problems with the learner's stage of self-direction

Although teachers of adult learners appreciate that there is a process involved in developing higher levels of self-direction, it does not always occur to them that their teaching level may mismatch their learner's current stage (*see* Chapter 5).[2]

Try asking yourself the following questions.

➤ Have I got a *dependent learner*? Do they request coaching with on-the-spot feedback and guidance? Are they happiest with lectures from experts and extensive handouts? Do they seem to ask frequently 'Is this in the exam?' Are they keen to find out the 'right answer' from you?

➤ Have I got an *interested learner*? Will they engage in guided discussion? Can they participate in goal setting and learning strategies? Do they sometimes ask you what books to read?

➤ Have I got an *involved learner*? Do they engage in discussions as an equal? Can they run and participate in seminars, doing background work and preparation for the group? Can they work alone (e.g. in projects)?

➤ Have I got a *self-directed learner*? Do they look to you as a supervisor of their work, someone who delegates tasks and can be consulted as need be? Do they have the study skills to analyse their own learning needs and devise a programme of study to address them?

Insight into this area may help you to explain a dysfunctional educational relationship. You are now one step away from adjusting your style to that of the learner (*see* Chapter 6).

Is there a mismatch of learning styles?

It helps to have insight into your own preferred learning activities, as this affects the way you teach. If you are engaged in a long-term teaching relationship, you could ask the learner to complete the Honey and Mumford learning styles questionnaire so that you are aware of each other's preferences.[3] You can then choose whether to challenge your learners by teaching against type, or match your teaching to their preferred style.

Perhaps the trainee who persistently fails to turn up on days when the training scheme is engaged in role play is a reflector–theorist without an activist bone in their body! Perhaps those learners chatting at the back of the class are activist–pragmatists who cannot see the relevance of this learning, or are bored with all the talk and no action. People who fill in evaluation forms stating that the pace of the day was too slow might be activists, and reflectors might find the same day too fast!

In shorter teaching programmes or one-off sessions, it is only possible to be aware of the variation in general terms, as it is not practicable to explore individual variations. Even so, your teaching strategy can take the likely variations into account.

Is the issue related to group work?

Probably the commonest clinical teaching setting is a small group, and all teachers will experience difficulties with the reactions and interactions of some members of the group.

A useful summary of behaviours within a group divides members into three categories (*see* Table 17.1). Behavioural styles include the following.[4]

➤ **The monopoliser**: enthusiastic, and often knowledgeable, this learner could be preventing others from contributing. Limit their domination of the discussion by summarising contributions and moving on, interjecting with yes or no answers and inviting others to contribute. Ask them to make written summaries of the group discussion. Split the group into smaller cells.

➤ **The rambler**: restrain contributions that cause diversions by asking direct questions of others. Address the problem head on (e.g. say 'That is interesting, but our point is . . .'. Defer until later (e.g. coffee time).

➤ **The eager beaver**: some learners try to answer every question. Acknowledge this help, but suggest that others should be asked for their views, or direct questions to others by name.

➤ **The conferrer**: ask yourself why this is happening. Do you need to change something you are doing? Stop talking and listen until they realise. Call them by name and draw them in with a direct question. Ask them whether they have anything to add to the discussion. Brief a co-facilitator to sit next to them to prevent a participant from being distracted.

➤ **The shy and timid**: allow time for their responses and value their contributions. Boost their confidence through social events. Protect them from mockery within the group.

➤ **The reticent**: Do they feel indifferent to the group or the task, or have they got something else on their mind? A non-participant may be unsure of the relevance of the task, or may be a reflector, or may be tired after being on call.

➤ **The superior**: Ensure that you have not got a false S4 learner (*see* Chapter 5). Encourage them to share their experience/expertise with the group. Use them to lead on tasks.

➤ **The complainer**: Control their fault finding by asking for specifics. Ask others in the group if they agree.

➤ **The clown**: Humour can be useful, but what is the constant joker really doing? Repeated irritating one-liners might be an attempt to upstage the teacher or to lighten a subject they find difficult. Compliment any serious contribution, and ask for the point behind the comment.

➤ **The arguer**: Antagonistic combatants like to score points. Avoid lengthy debate ('I think we will have to disagree'). Ask the group to comment – they will often criticise outlandish suggestions. Alternatively, take the person to one side and offer to 'help' if they have a problem.

Other participants can learn a lot from the varieties of opinions expressed in group work and the ways in which they are discussed, and they will also learn from how you deal with the situation. Only if one person's behaviour is seriously preventing others from learning, and after exhausting all other avenues, should you ask a group member to leave. There are some general principles for dealing with resistance in a group that are devised from the five beliefs of neurolinguistic programming (NLP), known as presuppositions of NLP.[5] Bear these ideas in mind when a learner is frustrating you!

1 The map is not the territory. Everyone has a different world view, and there is no one right model of the world.

2 Knowing other people's maps is useful in order to communicate with them effectively.

3 People make the best choices available to them at the time, given the possibilities and capabilities that they perceive are accessible to them.

4 Separate a person's behaviour from the intention behind it, and respond to the intention.

5 Resistance and objections are often communications about positive intentions that are not being met.

TABLE 17.1 Categories of challenging group members

The talker	Quiet and hesitant	Negative
The monopoliser	The shy and timid	The superior
The rambler	The reticent	The complainer
The eager beaver		The clown
The conferrer		The arguer

It is useful to presuppose that all behaviour is positively intended, and that negative behaviours are separate from the positive intent. Therefore identify the positive intent of the resistant person, and offer them other choices of behaviour to achieve the same positive intention.

NLP can also be used to help to plan learning needs using a simple model of goal achievement,[6] which is set out in four stages as follows.

1 Decide what you want.
2 Do something.
3 Notice what happens.
4 Be flexible – be prepared to change.

Is it an issue of time management?

If your learner persistently arrives after everyone else and can't seem to fit all the work into the day, first check that this is not due to a misunderstanding. Do they genuinely think the 8.30 am ward round starts at 9.00 am, or have they got conflicting commitments, such as a child to be dropped off at the nursery? This situation might be remedied by a simple renegotiation of working hours.

However, some learners never seem to cope well with meeting deadlines. They request extensions for project work, are late for meetings, their clinics overrun and their paperwork is left undone. This might be a time management problem. Discuss it and come to a joint understanding about why this issue has arisen. Sometimes learners have full, difficult lives, and the best you can be is supportive. Offer advice about priority setting, delegation, planning, organisation and not taking on too much.

WHY HEALTH PROFESSIONALS RUN INTO DIFFICULTIES: WIDER ISSUES

Apart from problems with educational processes, there are a number of other reasons why your learners may run into difficulties. You can categorise the various problems into four main areas:

1 personal conduct
2 professional conduct
3 competence and performance issues
4 health and sickness issues.

In any or all of these areas, adverse life events (see below) may have a profound influence.

Personal conduct issues that are not related to being a health professional

Examples of personal conduct issues include theft, fraud, assault, vandalism, rudeness, bullying, racial and sexual harassment, child pornography, drunkenness and serious traffic offences. The employer (or responsible body) should take the lead under its approved disciplinary procedures. Sometimes the police will be involved. In some situations regulatory bodies will be informed of an offence.

Normal procedure in the UK is that if a doctor in training is involved, the employer must inform both the doctor's postgraduate training/continuing professional development body (e.g. the deanery) and the trainee in writing at an early stage so that they may approach the training body for advice, particularly if there are any concerns that any allegations are as a result of professional issues and/or education and training difficulties. The training body will offer advice to the trainee to ensure that an agreed disciplinary procedure is followed, and advice on representation and pastoral support is given. In addition, national guidelines with regard to suspension are followed if this is appropriate. However, suspension is discouraged. Performance assessment services, such as the National Clinical Assessment Service (NCAS) and, for trainees, the postgraduate dean, must be consulted before this is carried out.

Professional conduct issues that are related to being a health professional

Examples of professional misconduct include inappropriate behaviour during clinical examinations, falsely claiming qualifications, plagiarism, research misconduct, failure to take consent properly, prescribing issues, improper relationships with patients, improper certification issues (e.g. the signing of cremation forms, sickness certification, passport forms), and breaches of confidentiality. Again, the employer (or responsible body) should take the lead under its approved disciplinary procedures. In some situations, regulatory bodies will be informed of an offence.

Any decision to involve the regulatory body is a very serious one for the professional involved, and this will be a joint decision between the employer and the postgraduate training/continuing professional development body (e.g. the deanery). Regulatory bodies generally recommend that approved procedures should be followed first at the local level, rather than everything being reported to national regulatory bodies at the earliest stage.

Competence and performance issues

Examples include a single serious clinical mistake, excessively slow surgical operating, poor clinical results (possibly found as a result of audit), persistent poor timekeeping, poor communication or English language skills, and repeated failure to attend educational events. Very basic problems can occur, including inability to take a history or examine a patient, and unsafe use of basic equipment. Most of these can be dealt with through the educational framework. An isolated serious mistake may happen to any practising healthcare professional, and usually does not reflect the overall competence of the individual.

Health and sickness issues

Depressive illness is common and sadly under-diagnosed. A few healthcare professionals will have a psychotic illness, and when this is uncontrolled it can be very serious and difficult to manage in the workplace. Alcohol- and drug-related problems occur. Healthcare professionals have physical illnesses just as others do, including multiple sclerosis, diabetes, arthritis and chronic respiratory diseases. Most of these problems can be successfully managed and the individual concerned restored to the workplace.

Adverse life events

Adverse life events may be a contributing factor to any of the above categories. People may experience horrendous adverse events which occurred outside of the workplace, and will often not volunteer such information. Ask about bereavements, severe illness, accidents, change of job, moving house, lack of family support, and so on. Sometimes healthcare professionals who work in one country have close family living in another, and may travel back and forth. This undoubtedly has an effect on the individual's personal and professional life.

You could use the following checklist when discussing adverse life events to highlight possible stressors and allow you to measure how severe each of them may be.

A score of 50 in a six-month period is considered to be stressful enough to cause illness.

Event	Score
Death of a parent	50
Death of a close relative	40
Loss of a parent through divorce	35
Death of a close friend	30
Parents having rows or in financial trouble	28
Serious health problems, surgery, pregnancy	25
Engagement or marriage	25
In trouble with the law	22
Unemployed, financial trouble	19
Break-up with boyfriend or girlfriend	19
Interviews or starting a new job	18
Sexual difficulties	18
'Not part of the crowd'	16
Lack of privacy	15
Driving test	15
College pressures, exams, deadlines	14
Concern about appearance, weight, identity	13
Recent move (home, school or college)	11
Lack of recognition	9
General feelings of frustration	6

A high score on this chart does not necessarily mean that a problem will arise, but it may provide an indication that solutions for reducing and managing stress should be identified.

Stress is cumulative. Sometimes it may be a small event that tips the balance following a series of major life events – 'the straw that broke the camel's back.'

RISK FACTORS THAT TRIGGER DIFFICULTIES FOR LEARNERS

Certain traits and situations will place your learners at risk of running into problems. Knowing these risk factors will alert you to when you need to be more vigilant with your learners, hopefully either pre-empting and thereby avoiding problems, or detecting them in their early stages.

Personality, behaviour and performance

Several personality characteristics can result in problems with behaviour and performance.[7] For example, macho or arrogant behaviour may be associated with individuals being unable to recognise their limitations, or when they are heading for problems. Such people tend towards authoritarianism and inappropriate behaviour. Although we might not be able to change people's personalities, it is often possible to detect and quantify unacceptable behaviours with multi-source feedback (MSF) (360 degree assessment) (*see* Chapter 13),[8] and to help to modify these behaviours with coaching, constructive feedback and, on occasion, sanctions.

Education and training

Healthcare education now puts more emphasis on communication skills (both with patients and with colleagues), on multi-disciplinary teamworking, and on appropriate attitudes and behaviours. Foreign healthcare professionals have difficulties when practising in a new country where there are differences in expected attitudes and behaviours.

A specific time to encounter difficulties is during the transition from student to practising professional.[9-11] Up to 1–2% of new doctors undergo remedial training and repeat all or part of their first year.[2]

Teamworking

Most of us work in teams, but how many of us work in supportive and effective teams? Working in a multi-disciplinary team is demanding. Good teams are rewarding to work in, result in less stress among their members, and provide a good and important sense of support. The dysfunctional team is the opposite of this. People become stressed and hate working. One member may ignore the wishes of others, and behave in an authoritarian and condescending way to other members, sometimes as a result of cultural attitudes.

Leadership (or lack of it)

Trainee healthcare professionals need education in leadership skills (*see* Chapter 19). This cannot be an optional extra.[12] There is growing evidence of links between the qualities of leaders and those of patient care.[2] Leaders should be able, intelligent, warm and friendly, benevolent, emotionally stable, and able to recognise limitations, delegate, predict and plan accordingly, and create a sense of justice. They should have good communication skills and integrity, and give people a sense of control. Unfortunately, some healthcare professionals in senior positions have few of these qualities!

Cognitive impairment

This term encompasses concerns about a person's memory, reasoning or decision making. It is uncommon, but senior healthcare professionals have run into problems of underperformance, and further investigations have revealed loss of short-term memory and dementia. Cognitive impairment may result from long-standing alcohol-related problems, certain neurological disorders, electroconvulsive therapy (ECT), severe head injury, stroke and coronary heart disease. It can be very difficult to diagnose cognitive impairment and to differentiate it from depression. Expert referral and assessment are necessary.

Organisational culture and climate

Organisational climate relates to staff perceptions of what it is like to work in the organisation.[13] Organisational culture includes climate, but is also about how to behave in the organisation, and leadership style and values. Compared with educational climate, where we have a variety of tools to use, and a growing literature (which has been summarised by Roff[14]), there seems to have been little research on organisational climate in the healthcare services. Ideally we would all like to work in an open, fair, friendly, sensitive and supportive culture, where we feel appreciated and valued. Working in a culture of institutional bullying and intimidation, scapegoating and poor leadership is stressful and should not be tolerated. Leaders who are ignorant, arrogant, dictatorial, hostile, boastful and generally not up to the job cause many problems – for example, less efficient working and high rates of staff absence and turnover, as people get fed up and look for opportunities to leave for other jobs where they feel more appreciated.

Heavy workload

Although the number of hours worked per week has slowly declined, the intensity and complexity of medical practice and other healthcare roles have greatly increased. Heavy workload, a 'long-hours' culture, lack of sleep and shift working can result in poor performance, and can make existing mental and physical health problems worse. A heavy workload may cause burnout. Shift working is especially risky at times when levels of sleepiness are high, such as between 1 am and 6 am, but in general it can have adverse physiological effects on the individual. Ensuring that there are proper timetabled breaks will help.

WAYS IN WHICH A PROBLEM MAY PRESENT

A UK medical performance assessment service has highlighted several early signs of doctors being in difficulty in terms of their education:[2]

➤ **the disappearing act:** not answering bleeps, 'disappearing', frequent sick leave, not attending teaching sessions, failure to turn up for work or learning events
➤ **low work rate:** slow in performing procedures, clerking patients and dictating letters, non-participation in group work, destructive group behaviour, not keeping up to date, failing to prepare for teaching, failure in exams
➤ **ward rage:** problems working in the team, shouting at colleagues, inability to give instructions to or take instructions from staff
➤ **rigidity:** low tolerance of uncertainty, difficulty in making priority decisions
➤ **bypass syndrome:** nurses and other colleagues avoid asking the doctor to do anything
➤ **career problems:** examination difficulty, disillusionment with medicine
➤ **insight failure:** rejection of constructive feedback, defensiveness, counter challenge.

Other signs of problems include the following:

➤ **inappropriate dress:** for example, T-shirts with logos, camouflage trousers and shirts when not in the Armed Services, and various items of traditional dress worn inappropriately
➤ **insufficient dress:** in particular, female professionals may not wear enough to maintain their modesty. Remember that inappropriate or strange dress may be a presentation of psychiatric illness
➤ **body piercings:** for example, multiple ear, tongue, lip and eyebrow piercings, and piercings on various other parts of the body
➤ **hairstyles:** some professionals have weird and wonderful hairstyles more appropriate to a rock star
➤ **tattoos:** patients may find visible tattoos offputting
➤ **smelly dirty individuals:** some are obviously unwashed, smell of body odour and wear smelly trainers – this is not what patients would expect
➤ **bizarre email addresses:** mistress.megadoc@doctors.org.uk and the.greatest@ heartofengland.nhs.uk are not real email addresses, but are illustrations of those that are actually used.

Many of the signs of individuals in difficulty are now picked up by MSF (*see* Chapter 13).

In many cases, individuals will have multiple problems, not just one. A study of 123 consequential referrals of psychiatrists in difficulty showed that most of them had multiple problems.[15] Often an individual who was referred with a performance or communication problem turned out to have experienced several recent adverse life events and/or a major health problem. Often all of the underlying problems are unknown to the organisation or individual who has picked up upon the initial concern, or who is referring the healthcare professional in difficulty for help or investigation.

WHAT SHOULD WE DO IN PRACTICE? A SIX-POINT PLAN

When learners are in difficulty, you should follow a set procedure. This may need to be adapted for your local services. However, an example for doctors in difficulty is provided in Figure 17.2. The process, in more general terms, is summarised below.

Phase 1: the referral

Referral to the training/postgraduate professional development organisation may be made by letter, telephone, face-to-face contact or email (which we discourage unless complete confidentiality can be ensured). Information is read, and a decision is made to either accept the referral or suggest other ways of dealing with the situation. For example, the police or the individual's professional regulatory body may be a more appropriate route for some situations.

Phase 2: meeting the individual

Meet with the individual concerned. An introduction is essential, including an explanation that this process is intended to help the person, and is *not* a telling off or disciplinary meeting. Ask the individual to tell their story. Rather than have an unstructured and often rambling conversation, structure the conversation. Frame the meeting, and say that after the introductions you will be asking about the situation in four areas as follows:

1 **the career history** from undergraduate to the present time, including the person's career aims
2 **the present problem** as the person perceives it
3 **health issues and adverse life events** (see above), using the adverse life events framework if necessary
4 **the plan of action proposed** – this may be to offer a diagnosis and a plan of actions to help, or more frequently you will need to obtain further information, and meet again.

Phase 3: a provisional diagnosis

Make a provisional diagnosis of what you think is the problem. Often you will need further information and other assessments in order to clarify the situation. For example, you might ask for a consultant-led occupational health assessment, a communication skills assessment, trainer reports, a further MSF exercise, and so on. You should then arrange to meet again to review all of this.

Phase 4: a case discussion

When you meet again with the individual with the extra information, you should explain all of the findings and make a decision on what to do. Sometimes no action is needed, but often you will need to put in place further training of some kind and/or move the healthcare professional to another post. Career advice and sometimes career counselling may be necessary. Rarely you may be required to advise suspension, or even to advise that the individual leaves their training programme and/or post altogether. Very rarely you will need to refer to the professional regulatory body. Before doing this you must discuss the case at the highest level within your local institution/organisation. Once the referral has gone in it is unstoppable, and it is often unpredictable what actions will be taken. So think very carefully.

Hopefully the individual concerned will agree with the advised course of action, which needs to be clearly set out.

Phase 5: the review

Usually you will arrange to see the individual again so that the implementation and success of the action plan can be assessed. Has improvement occurred?

Phase 6: follow-up

Sometimes you will need to arrange a longer-term follow-up of certain individuals who find themselves in difficulty, in order to keep them on track. Sometimes this is because of illness, or a requirement from their regulatory body, or because they do not make the required levels of progress.

This process is presented diagrammatically in Figure 17.2.

SOME KEY CONCEPTS TO CONSIDER WHEN DEALING WITH PEOPLE IN DIFFICULTY

Remember the following concepts, and don't take everything at face value. A health problem may present as a performance issue, and vice versa. If you do not establish the real problem, you will not solve anything. The six-step problem-solving approach might help (*see* Chapter 13).

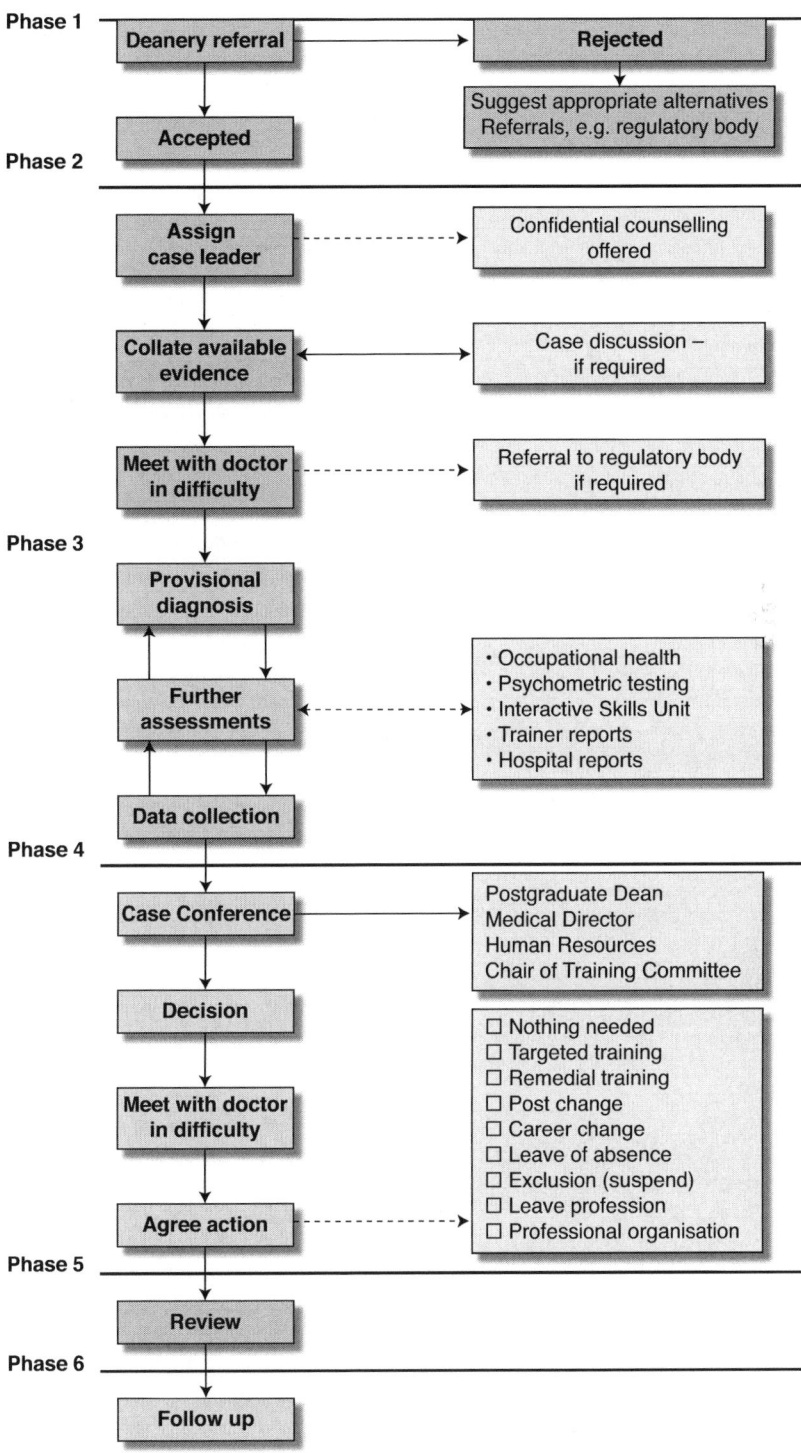

FIGURE 17.2

Many problems can be resolved at local level. The principles of establishing and using the facts (and not opinions), constructive feedback and setting targets for improvement, and following these through, will work well in most cases.

Why has this happened?
Sometimes problems may not be immediately apparent and may be multiple. Therefore, when faced with a learner whom you believe is either heading for or already in difficulty, consider the following points.

➤ **Is it the trainee, the trainer, the job or the interplay between these?** Define why difficulties have arisen. Asking this basic question may be very useful in clarifying where you need to focus. Sometimes it is the trainer or the organisation, and the individual in difficulty is a 'symptom' of greater and more fundamental difficulties in the organisation. At other times, problems may occur due to a personality clash between learner and teacher.

➤ **Does the person need career advice?** Are they in the wrong career? Many sources of career advice are now available through the postgraduate organisations and their websites. Approach the local clinical tutor in the first instance, who may be able to help, or who may pass you on to a regional adviser or the postgraduate organisation. You may identify people who hate healthcare and who are in the wrong career.

➤ **Does the person have other problems such as stress, physical or mental illness, etc.?** Everyone should be registered with a general practitioner, and you should ensure that this is the case. Where sickness absence or suspected illness does give cause for concern, or the individual has unfortunately developed a serious communicable disease or disability, the opinion of a consultant physician in occupational medicine is essential. Remember patient confidentiality here (the person in difficulty being the patient). Such a referral must be labelled *private and confidential* and not sent via email with multiple copies. This is confidential medical information. You are not the person's doctor, so leave it to those who are.

Working with senior consultants in occupational medicine who are experienced in dealing with healthcare professionals in difficulty, with time to meet and to discuss ideas and policies, is immensely beneficial, especially for the individuals who are experiencing problems.

Early diagnosis and tackling of problems
If you are involved in managing an individual in difficulty, the principles listed below will be helpful.

➤ **Do it now:** Tackle the problem when it occurs, not at the end of the placement or not at all.

➤ **Find out the facts:** Don't jump to conclusions. Obtain information from all sides.

➤ **Share the problem:** Don't do it all on your own, but get advice from others (other trainers, educational supervisors, your specialty tutor, your clinical tutor, the training programme director, the chair of your training committee, regional advisers, the local, regional or national healthcare organisation and/or postgraduate training/continuing professional development organisation). Expert assessments and opinions about occupational health and communication skills will prove really helpful.

➤ **Explain the problem:** Discuss the problem constructively with the individual concerned, and plan how to get back on course. Sometimes no one has sat down with the individual and explained what the difficulty is, and how this may be put right. Sometimes people will say that this was the first time that anyone had mentioned to them that they have a communication skills or teamworking problem.

➤ **Give support:** Appropriate encouragement and positive feedback do work.

The role of the employer/contracting organisation

Healthcare professionals will always have an employer. This may be the healthcare organisation or the university. Those in career grades may be employed by the health-care service or be self-employed healthcare professionals. Legally, the employer must take the lead in all four areas of problems. Employers will have procedures laid down for discipline, performance and sickness issues.

It is very important that those responsible for training know about problems when one of their trainees is involved. In order to deal with the issue of confidentiality, the healthcare organisation that employs a trainee should inform him or her that the post-graduate training organisation may be approached for advice. What happens next will depend on the types of problems that are encountered and their seriousness.

GETTING BACK ON TRACK: GUIDING PRINCIPLES

The National Clinical Assessment Service (NCAS)[16] has described 11 key principles for handling performance concerns. These are as follows.

1 Patient safety must be the primary consideration.
2 Healthcare organisations are responsible for developing policies and procedures to recognise performance concerns early and act swiftly to address those concerns.
3 Policies for handling performance concerns should be circulated to all healthcare practitioners.
4 Avoid unnecessary or inappropriate exclusions of practitioners.
5 Separate investigation from decision making.
6 Staff and managers should understand the factors that may contribute to perfor-mance concerns.
7 Performance procedures should contribute to the organisational programme for clinical governance.
8 Good human resources practice will help to prevent performance problems.
9 Healthcare practitioners who work in isolated settings may require additional support.
10 Individual healthcare practitioners are responsible for maintaining a good standard of practice.
11 There must be commitment to equality and diversity.

BACK-ON-TRACK FRAMEWORK

The NCAS[17] has outlined seven guiding principles for helping professionals who are in difficulty. These are as follows.

1 **Clinical governance and patient safety:** Patient safety must come first.
2 **A single framework guiding individual programmes:** Use of a framework must encompass common principles, which are applicable in different specialties and for different grades.
3 **A comprehensive approach:** Identify and deal with problems comprehensively, identifying all of the issues, dealing with the needs of the individual and the organisation, and keeping the need to protect patient safety as a primary concern. Communication skills are often a problem, so work closely with communication skills teachers to help to identify and improve communication skills in many of those individuals who are in difficulty.
4 **Fairness, transparency, confidentiality and patient consent:** You must be fair and open about what you do. The confidentiality of the person in difficulty needs to be protected. Copy letters to the organisations involved, to occupational health (where applicable), and to the person in difficulty so that they know exactly what has been said and why. However, there is a guiding principle here about the need to know, so such information should only be given to those helping in the process. Patients need to be properly informed if they are being seen by an individual who is on a return-to-work programme. Fairness also involves being aware of and practising fairness in terms of the legislation on equality of opportunity with regard to age, gender, ethnicity, religion, sexual orientation and disability.
5 **Ongoing and constant support:** This is essential. Support for some individuals in difficulty may be necessary for several years, sticking with it despite setbacks. In certain cases, individuals may be 'on the books' for over 10 years. Good progress can still occur even after this time, but it can be a long hard journey with considerable setbacks on the way. In such cases the remedial training team and the healthcare organisation can be under considerable load. Often such teams need breaks from training after dealing with an individual in difficulty, as remedial training can put considerable stress on the whole team. You may need to be aware of and recognise this as a significant issue.
6 **Success and failure:** Although you hope that dealing with the problems of individuals in difficulty will help them to succeed and get back on track, this is not always the case. Think of what to do if a programme of return to work does not succeed, and how to spell out what is to happen if objectives are not achieved. Sometimes, for those individuals with severe physical or mental illness, despite all measures to cope, the only solution may be an early retirement on medical grounds. Here obviously the continuing involvement and close collaboration of a senior consultant in occupational medicine is essential. On rare occasions, in other situations, where the individual is felt to pose a danger to patients, a referral to the appropriate regulatory body will be appropriate.

   If you are dealing with individuals in difficulty, you must acknowledge that you cannot succeed in every case. You also need support from your professional organisation.
7 **Local resolution drawing on local and national expertise:** Use local procedures first. Sharing your experiences is also very valuable at the local and/or regional level. People need to be trained at local level in managing poor performance, so that they know what to look out for, what to do, and when and where to refer on for help if necessary.

FUNDING

Who pays for the person to be re-trained? This is a very difficult issue.

For those who are trainees and who are already in approved training programmes, it is easier, as the postgraduate training organisation will keep some posts for such eventualities.

For healthcare professionals who are employed or contracted in career posts, some healthcare organisations are willing to fund or part-fund a return-to-work programme, including help with courses, for a specific period of time according to a programme of training and assessment. A 2006 UK review recommended that there should be a funding contribution from the employing healthcare organisation.[18] However, in practice this varies enormously. For certain professionals there can be a considerable problem of locum costs for backfilling the work of the individual while they are away re-training.

The situation is dire for individuals who are unemployed, who are not trainees, or who have been suspended or erased from the professional register for several years. However, they may expect to be given a job immediately. Often such individuals are in considerable difficulty in many areas, have a chaotic life situation, are in debt, and are unable to fund their re-training. The suggestion that such individuals should take out a loan, when they may already be in considerable debt and have no creditworthiness at all, is not viable. A clear policy and ring-fenced funding are required to help to rehabilitate such desperate individuals. Remember that not everyone is remediable (see below).

REMEDIABILITY WITH REGARD TO DOCTORS IN DIFFICULTY

Remediability refers to whether an individual's problems may be successfully addressed and their career put back on track, or whether the prognosis is so poor that other measures need to be considered. In the area of remediation, we need to know what we may take on with the hope of successful remediation back into practice, or whether we need to consider other measures such as referral to the regulatory organisation or advice on resignation or retirement from the post. Can we predict how well a person in difficulty will respond? To some extent the answer is yes. Here is a classification that you might find useful, which is partly derived from discussions at the Network of Expertise Group at the NCAS.

Capacity to learn

Some individuals may have lost the capacity to learn, perhaps due to brain injury, various neurological disorders or the development of cognitive impairment. Some of these cases represent really sad situations. Without capacity to learn, the prognosis is poor.

Knowledge or skill deficit

If a specific area of knowledge or skill deficit has been identified, and the healthcare professional recognises this fact, has insight and is willing to learn, focused training in that area will help. Such a deficit may respond well to specific training. Obviously it is essential to monitor progress in order to demonstrate that improvement has occurred. Here the prognosis is good.

Arousal and motivation

Some individuals may be too bored or too overwhelmed to work and learn effectively. These are problems with workload. This may be due to an overwhelming clinical workload and sleep deprivation sapping any motivation to work. However, in some cases healthcare professionals seem to have a lot of time off, appear bored and uninterested in their work, and take a lot of motivating to do anything. A change of post, inspirational trainers and role models, and regular meetings with the supervisor may help. The prognosis here is good.

Distraction

Many individuals are distracted – sometimes by health issues, but more often by adverse life events outside of work. These include bereavement, family illness, financial problems, break-up of relationships, and so on. Many people have multiple problems. Such difficulties often present as problems in workplace performance. If you can sort out what are the real problems underlying this, you stand a really good chance of helping the individual to get back on track. If you can do this, the prognosis is good.

Alienation

Once the individual is alienated, angry, has a feeling of injustice and lacks belief that they have a problem which can be helped, the prognosis is very poor indeed. Anger and hostility significantly obstruct help offered to the individual. For example, an individual who feels that they have been incorrectly singled out and victimised by their regulatory body may find it very difficult to recognise areas for improvement and to construct a personal development plan. Time and energy may be spent pursuing senior or government involvement for support, when this time might be better spent trying to improve clinical activities. Here the prognosis is very poor.

Lack of insight

In some ways, lack of insight may have features of alienation (see above), but not always. However, lack of insight is the most serious problem of the lot. An individual who lacks insight into their problematic behaviours or attitudes or their knowledge or skill deficits has a very poor prognosis.

Behaviours and their prognosis: are they treatable?

It is almost impossible to change personality. However, we may be able to change behaviours – but not in all cases. Feedback on performance, with good evidence to back it up (e.g. from MSF) is the key to achieving behaviour change. For example, individuals have been helped to work better within a team, and understand how to relate to other team members through the use of evidence from a MSF exercise, role-play sessions with experts on clinical communication, and constructive feedback on such behaviours. Continued monitoring of the individual's performance, using MSF in many cases, produces an acceptable level of performance which is sustained in the longer term.

There are pre-conditions for changing behaviours. The individual needs to be sufficiently intelligent, stable and perceptive, and have insight into their problems. As noted earlier, lack of insight is a considerable problem in this area, as is a history of previous unsuccessful attempts to change, and not being motivated to change. Unless the individual sees a reason to change and really wants to do so, it will be very difficult to achieve success.

Summary

So in summary, here are the categories of problems and their respective prognoses.

Capacity to learn	May have reached limit	Prognosis poor
Learning deficit	More training will often help	Prognosis good
Arousal and motivation	Too bored or too overwhelmed	Prognosis good
Distraction	Problems elsewhere (e.g. health)	Prognosis good
Alienation	Deep-rooted feeling of injustice	Prognosis very poor
Lack of insight	No acceptance of a problem	Prognosis very poor

Consider whether an individual's problems are remediable or not. In many situations it is worth trying to help. However, in some cases, after the various initiatives have really not worked, it is essential to conduct a re-assessment of what you are doing and whether it is advisable to continue. In some cases the better option is to withdraw, to inform the individual's director or manager of this opinion, and perhaps to offer advice on retirement or change of job, or consider notification to the appropriate regulatory body.

REFERENCES

1 Luft J. *Group Processes: an introduction to group dynamics.* Palo Alto, CA: National Press Books; 1970.

2 Grow GO. Teaching learners to be self-directed. *Adult Educ Quarterly.* 1996; **41:** 125–49.

3 Honey P, Mumford A. *Using Your Learning Styles.* Maidenhead: Peter Honey; 1986.

4 Allery L. *Dealing with Challenging Group Members. Two sides of A4.* Number 4. Cardiff: School of Postgraduate Studies, University of Wales College of Medicine; 1998.

5 Walker L. *Consulting with NLP.* Oxford: Radcliffe Medical Press; 2002.

6 Alder H. *NLP for Managers: how to achieve excellence at work.* London: Piatkus; 1996.

7 National Clinical Assessment Authority. *Understanding Performance Difficulties in Doctors. An NCAA report.* London: National Clinical Assessment Authority; 2004.

8 Whitehouse AB, Hassell A, Bullock A *et al.* 360 degree assessment (multisource feedback) of UK trainee doctors: field testing of TAB. *Med Teacher.* 2007; **29:** 171–6.

9 Bligh J. The first year of doctoring: still a survival exercise. *Med Educ.* 2002; **36:** 2–3.

10 Wall D, Bolshaw A, Carolan J. From undergraduate medical education to pre-registration house officer year: how prepared are students? *Med Teacher.* 2006; **28:** 435–9.

11 Farrah K. Time to review prescribing in hospitals by pre-registration house officers. *Pharm J.* 2002; **268:** 136.

12 Spurgeon P. *Leadership Education for all Doctors: no longer an optional extra.* Short presentation 7G/SC4 presented at AMEE Conference, 27 August 2007, Trondheim. http://amee. org

13 Scott T, Mannion R, Marshall M *et al.* Does organisational culture influence health care performance? A review of the evidence. *J Health Serv Res Policy.* 2003; **8:** 105–17.

14 Roff S. Education environment: a bibliography. *Med Teacher.* 2005: **27:** 353–7.

15 O'Leary D. *Performance Concerns in Psychiatrists.* Poster 4P/P8 presented at AMEE Conference, 27 August 2007, Trondheim. http://amee.org

16 National Clinical Assessment Service. *Handling Concerns about the Performance of Healthcare*

Professionals: principles of good practice. London: National Clinical Assessment Service; 2006.

17 National Clinical Assessment Service. *Back on Track: restoring doctors and dentists to safe professional practice.* Framework document. London: National Clinical Assessment Service; 2006.

18 Chief Medical Officer. *Good Doctors, Safer Patients.* London: Department of Health; 2006.

CHAPTER 18

Providing supervision and support

The first part of this chapter focuses on how to be a good mentor, educational supervisor, careers counsellor or coach. You might be all of these to several people, or more than one of these to the same person. These roles may overlap and sometimes conflict.

We then look at the special considerations for teaching and supporting learners with special needs, and at aspects of pastoral care.

HOW TO BE A GOOD MENTOR, EDUCATIONAL SUPERVISOR, CAREERS COUNSELLOR OR COACH

There are many overlaps between all of these terms, but the roles of each are distinct. The terms are all part of common parlance, and those in authority may believe that they have the skills by virtue of their position, not understanding all of the implications of the role or the total responsibility that they carry.

Sometimes one individual is expected to be a mentor, educational supervisor, line manager and careers counsellor to the same person, and conflicts of interest can arise. It is difficult for everyone involved if an individual who is acting as the careers counsellor has authority over the health professional client and the ability to change their work circumstances in a negative way. The 'client' is unlikely to trust the independence of the counsellor, and the counsellor may act on their acquired insider knowledge on a future occasion.

BEING A SKILLED MENTOR

A mentor helps the person who is being mentored (here termed a 'mentee') to realise their potential by acting as a trusted senior counsellor and experienced guide on personal, professional and educational matters. As a mentor you should agree learning objectives with your mentee and subsequently guide them as they address their educational needs, help them to identify their strengths and weaknesses, explore options with them, act as a challenger, encourage reflection and provide motivation.

Your relationship with your mentee should be one of mutual trust and respect in a supportive yet challenging relationship. You should not be involved in promotion, remuneration, assessments or appraisals of your mentee, as this may undermine your relationship if there is a conflict of interest, and preclude you from being non-judgemental – a cornerstone of mentoring.

Mentoring is 'the process by which an experienced, highly regarded, empathic person (the mentor) guides another individual (the mentee) in the development and re-examination of their own ideas, learning, and personal and professional development. The mentor, who often, but not necessarily, works in the same organisation or field as the mentee, achieves this by listening and talking in confidence to the mentee.'[1] The emphasis is on the mentor helping the mentee to develop their own thinking and find their own way, not on teaching the mentee new skills or acting as a patron to ease the mentee's career path by special favours.

In order to be a successful mentor you should be well matched with and chosen by your mentee, and you should both be willing participants – mentoring should be voluntary. You will need ongoing support.

Start by agreeing ground rules with regard to confidentiality, commitment, the duration and frequency of sessions, location, the purpose, personal boundaries and how or whether you will record your meetings. Clarify the objectives and outcomes that you both want to address. A common framework that is used for mentoring follows three stages:

1 Exploration: the mentor listens and prompts the mentee with questions.
2 New understanding: the mentor listens and challenges the mentee, recognises the strengths and weaknesses of the ideas, shares experiences, establishes priorities, identifies development needs, and gives information and supportive feedback.
3 Action planning: the mentor encourages new ways of thinking, helps the mentee to reach a solution, agrees goals and decides on action plans.

Characteristics of a good mentor[1,2]

A good mentor:
➤ is committed
➤ is honest and trustworthy
➤ is non-judgemental
➤ has good interpersonal skills
➤ is patient
➤ is open and approachable
➤ is knowledgeable, experienced and wise
➤ is confident
➤ has good contacts
➤ is respected
➤ is empathetic
➤ is enthusiastic and encouraging.

A mentor and mentee may have different backgrounds, and the differences may provoke a cross-fertilisation of ideas and a general improvement of understanding of the healthcare service from another's point of view. People learn best in environments that are directly related to the learning that is taking place. The mentoring session is the bridge between theory and reality. It may be an opportunity to reinforce or analyse what learning took place after actually doing a new task, when a different perspective can be brought into play in order to gain the most benefit. The mentor and mentee should define what competency the mentee wishes to develop under each of the learning objectives they agree as components of the purpose of the mentoring taking place. For instance, if the purpose of a mentoring session was for the mentee to understand how to manage their workload better, the competences that the mentor and mentee should be reflecting on might be delegation, prioritisation and information technology skills.

Box 18.1 lists the problems that can arise in the mentor/mentee relationship, and how they may be overcome.

BOX 18.1 Overcoming possible problems arising in a mentor/mentee relationship

- Time commitment: assess it accurately and plan for it.
- Conflict of interests if the mentor is the mentee's 'line manager': define the relationship, and if trust is impossible, find a different mentor/mentee match.
- Strained relationship between mentor and mentee: agree boundaries to get the right balance between empathy and intimacy.
- The 'halo' effect: both should be aware that the learner may attribute a 'halo' to the mentor, whose opinions may be seen as absolute answers. Discuss and defuse this tendency.
- Other colleagues being jealous of the close relationship between mentor and mentee: beware of the mentee being accused of getting an unfair amount of attention and support, and try not to let your relationship fuel resentment.
- Criticism of the mentee by the mentor: both should be aware of the sensitivities of the mentee to any criticism, and take the utmost care with formal and informal, verbal and non-verbal feedback. Discuss problems analytically without involving personalities.
- Gender difference leading to inappropriate sexual attraction: take care to act professionally at all times.
- Dislike by one or each of the other: liking each other is essential. Discontinue such a mentor/mentee relationship.

The ABC model of mentoring[3]

A   Achieve a relationship.
B   Boil the problem down: formative and supportive roles.
C   Challenge the person to change or cope.

Mentoring is a developmental process for the mentee,[4-6] who should gain from:
- improved performance that can be evaluated back in the workplace and lead to more defined objectives at the next mentoring session
- new insights and perspectives from another individual or professional point of view
- increased confidence
- improved interpersonal skills
- an increase in personal influencing skills

➤ knowledge and skills
➤ having their perceptions and beliefs challenged
➤ enjoying the challenges of change
➤ an open and flexible attitude to learning
➤ overcoming setbacks and obstacles
➤ developing values and an ethical perspective
➤ increasing their listening, analytical and problem-solving skills
➤ conscious reflection that enhances learning.

Learning contract for mentor/mentee

You might formalise your relationship as mentor to a mentee by drawing up a learning contract (*see* Box 18.2).[4]

BOX 18.2 A mentor/mentee learning contract

Mentor   Name: Mentee   Name:

       Position: Position:

       Signature: Signature:

Purpose of mentorship:
Date mentorship began:
Agreed length of each session:
Agreed timetable:
Areas to be covered in sessions:
Review period:
Mentor comments:
Mentee comments:
Satisfied/not satisfied:

BEING A GOOD SUPERVISOR

Educational supervision

An educational supervisor works with the learner to develop and facilitate an educational plan that addresses their educational needs. Ideally, educational supervision should be focused on educational development and be separate from supervision of clinical practice or remedial help for under-performance. However, this is rarely possible in practice, and an educational supervisor usually has multiple responsibilities for a trainee. They may be expected to give support, facilitate education and training, supervise educational progress, supervise clinical work, provide and coordinate service-based training, provide support for formal educational programmes, provide pastoral and careers counselling, and perhaps represent the employer.

The educational supervisor should agree a structured personal educational plan with the learner, dependent on the learner's needs and aspirations. The supervisor will usually maintain an overview of the learner's performance and career progress.

The role of the educational supervisor[7] (also *see* Box 18.3) is to provide:

➤ professional and personal support for the learner
➤ facilitation of education and training
➤ supervision of the learner's educational progress
➤ supervision of the trainee's clinical work as appropriate
➤ coordinated service-based training
➤ support for a formal educational programme
➤ pastoral and careers counselling as required
➤ good employer practice – ensuring a clear job description/training prospectus for each post (if the learner is an employee).

In other countries (e.g. the USA and Canada) and in certain professions (e.g. nursing), a similar role may be undertaken by preceptors, who provide clinical and professional support to facilitate learning.[8] Preceptors may only be used for the first few years after qualification to ensure appropriate support and development of new workers.

BOX 18.3 The role of the educational supervisor

An educational supervisor should:
• meet with the learner early in the post and help with the induction to the post
• agree the aims and objectives for learning in the post
• construct the learning agreement with the learner
• give feedback on progress to the learner
• discuss career aims and the training programme
• assess the learner at the end of the post on their learning objectives
• give feedback to the teacher on the training posts and programmes (if appropriate).

Training programmes are often 'trainee led', so your trainees should approach you and be proactive in organising meetings. However, it is useful for you to make your availability known to learners to facilitate them arranging meetings and asking for advice and/or support when needed.

Clinical supervision

Clinical supervision includes a 'formative' function, which is about the educative process of developing skills, a 'restorative' process, where professionals are given supportive help, and a 'normative' component, which covers the managerial and quality control aspects of professional practice. In the USA and Canada, clinical supervisors, particularly of nurses, may be known as 'field' or 'ward preceptors', and for medics, senior physicians who supervise the clinical work of juniors may be known as 'faculty.'

Clinical supervisors should encourage *experiential learning*, taking learners all the way round the Kolb cycle.[9]

➤ Do (concrete experience).
➤ Review (reflective observation).
➤ Learn (theory building, abstract ideas).
➤ Apply (active experimentation, the testing of ideas).

➤ Do.
➤ etc.

Effective learning builds on experience if it is to make sense in an organisational context and be relevant to health service needs.

Being an effective careers counsellor

Careers counselling enables people to recognise and utilise their resources to manage career-related problems and make career-related decisions. Ideally, careers counselling builds on careers advice or guidance, appraisal and assessment, and pastoral support. It includes the recognition and analysis of a person's strengths and weaknesses with respect to available career options, and should incorporate personal and professional development. To make a rational career choice, people need *careers information* – that is, the facts about career opportunities, including the number and types of post available at a particular level and in a particular specialty, and details of the qualifications and training necessary. *Careers guidance* is more personal and directive, and provides advice within the context of the opportunities that are available for those who have not made a career decision, or who have decided on their career goal but are unaware of the best way of achieving it. A learner may use one or all of the sources of help, depending on their individual needs.

Most health professionals will not have the skills necessary to be an effective careers counsellor without further training. A postgraduate diploma in careers counselling is a lengthy course. The counselling skills that are used in clinical work are helpful, but cannot be automatically extrapolated and applied to a careers counselling situation. In order to be an effective careers counsellor, you should:

➤ be non-judgemental
➤ transmit unconditional positive regard to the person who is being counselled
➤ know yourself well, so that you can recognise your own prejudices
➤ understand that your own preferences may not match those of others
➤ be aware of the range of opportunities for career development
➤ know from where individuals can seek more specialist career advice
➤ have sufficient insight and intuition to be able to understand the cause of difficulties within jobs or circumstances
➤ challenge the other person's restrictive attitudes, beliefs or behaviour
➤ give direct feedback on unconscious behaviour and challenge illogicalities or inconsistencies.

The various stages of careers counselling involve getting people to think through the following sequence of challenges.

➤ Who am I and where am I now?
➤ How satisfied am I with my career and my life?
➤ What changes would I like to make?
➤ How can I make them happen?
➤ What can I do if I don't get what I want?

Careers counselling is *not* about giving advice, but about encouraging people to reflect on their own situation and find their own solutions. Giving advice might:

➤ absolve individuals from taking responsibility
➤ be wrong for a particular individual
➤ be too superficial – decisions made through reflection and experience are more likely to be maintained and be satisfying
➤ result in the counsellor being blamed if the advice turns out to be wrong
➤ be a pet preference or personal prejudice of the counsellor.

People need careers counselling when they are:
➤ dissatisfied with their current job or career prospects
➤ unable to solve their career dilemma by themselves, although they do usually have the resources to do so
➤ unable to think clearly about their career and need to talk things through with an independent and non-judgemental person
➤ not responding to the usual motivators at work
➤ unaware of the consequences of their poor performance or behaviour at work
➤ engaging in self-deprecating behaviour at work
➤ unaware of their talents and strengths at work.

BEING A COMPETENT COACH

Coaching involves a combination of psychology, business and communication skills. It consists of a partnership between coach and 'client', which aims to clarify the client's goals for work and life, and to plan how to achieve those goals. The interactive relationship enhances the potential and performance of the person who is being coached to a greater extent than seemed possible when they were functioning on their own. Much of the culture of coaching healthcare professionals has been modelled from sports coaching. Sometimes the coach is brought in as an external catalyst, while at other times an in-house manager or senior professional will coach professionals at any stage of their career. Coaching is sometimes confined to learning a specific skill for a future event (e.g. a job interview or presentation at a conference), while at other times it might be focused on the person as a whole, to help them to progress more quickly with their professional and career development. Every coaching situation is different, as each coach has their own particular style of working, and each client has individual circumstances and is at a particular stage in their life.

A professional or 'executive' coach generally has a minimum of five years' experience as a coach, and a professional qualification (e.g. clinical psychology, occupational psychology, diploma in counselling, master practitioner in neurolinguistic programming or psychotherapy). Such an experienced coach will have expert knowledge of leadership and management behaviour, know about the theory and practice of organisational behaviour and human psychology, be accredited to use personality profile testing and other personal assessment techniques, and have many interpersonal skills.

Coaching provides an opportunity to focus on an individual's unique learning and development needs, and to set out a programme to meet those needs. Coaching usually starts with an evaluation of the individual's current effectiveness and their use of time and priorities. A good coach will:
➤ encourage the learner to reflect on how to build on their strengths to change their current situation

➤ help the learner to overcome self-imposed limitations that are preventing them from progressing as they might otherwise do

➤ build positive attitudes and behaviour in the learner – someone with a positive attitude and fewer skills is more likely to develop further than another person with more skills but a negative attitude

➤ be a successful motivator

➤ be supportive

➤ establish a good rapport with the learner

➤ give constructive feedback

➤ set clear objectives

➤ stretch and challenge the learner

➤ encourage the learner to solve problems and make changes by him- or herself

➤ be analytical rather than critical

➤ depersonalise the problems discussed in coaching sessions by focusing on facts, outcomes and performance rather than personalities or style

➤ have sufficient experience and expertise in the particular skill that the learner is trying to acquire.

The development of self-awareness and insight that results from coaching should lead to lasting change. The outcomes of coaching may vary depending on the circumstances of the person who is being coached. For example, they may tackle their job more effectively and enthusiastically, having clearer objectives, or they may reorganise or change their systems or situation at work so that they perform better, or they may re-evaluate their career and decide to find a different job:

> During the coaching, people gradually connect with their true ambitions and identify what steps are needed to achieve them. They gain more control of their lives and feel less tossed about by events. The feedback we get later from clients confirms that this is truly the case.[10]

A typical framework for a coaching session might be as follows:

➤ hear what has happened since the last meeting

➤ agree the topics to work on

➤ agree what should be achieved by the end of the session

➤ agree the priorities if there are too many issues

➤ undertake problem solving for each priority issue

➤ discuss what is the issue and its importance

➤ discuss what has been tried already

➤ agree what would be an ideal state

➤ debate what is preventing the ideal state from happening now

➤ establish the extent to which the individual is preventing the ideal state from being achieved

➤ explore the options for resolving the problem

➤ discuss what skills are needed for the preferred option

➤ agree the strategy and target(s)

➤ select appropriate training methods

➤ timetable training realistically.

POTENTIAL FOR ROLE CONFLICT

Some of the above responsibilities might overlap. Sometimes the qualities that are needed for one role can be used to great advantage in another. The roles of career counsellor and appraiser are one example.

Potentially, however, there is a risk of conflict of interest. You must tease out your responsibilities and decide which hat you are wearing at any one time if you are to provide effective support for learners who are looking to you for advice. For example, how does your responsibility as line manager interact with your responsibility as educational supervisor? As a line manager you may wish to keep a learner away from patients on the grounds of patient safety, but as an educational supervisor you realise that supervised experience is what they need in order to improve.

Information that is exchanged during mentoring sessions may have implications for your line manager or assessor roles. How confidential can such a relationship be? Learners may not regard you as a route through which they can explore their fears and worries if they have concerns that you will also be responsible for their assessments, or have some power over their ability to earn a living.

You can tell if things are not working out in any supervisory or support role if any of the features listed in Box 18.4 apply.

BOX 18.4 Features of a supervisory or support role
that is not working out well

- The mentor talks without stopping.
- The learner is unable to confide in his educational supervisor because he knows he will soon need a reference.
- A supervisor consistently puts service needs above an individual's training needs.
- The careers counsellor often tells learners how he or she managed his or her own career.
- The coach undermines others' self-confidence and self-esteem.

ADAPTING YOUR TEACHING STYLE AND HABITS FOR LEARNERS WITH DISABILITIES

An effective teacher adapts their delivery to meet the needs of their learners. Consider learners in different groups, particularly how to overcome challenges relating to learners with special needs. To treat people equally is not necessarily to treat them fairly. Since people are so different, 'equal treatment probably means injustice for most.'[11] Consider your teaching delivery so that you meet their learning styles or capabilities and do not disadvantage them more than is necessary.

Good teachers will recognise the negative effects of 'singling out' learners for special attention. It requires great sensitivity to address difference without making it more of a barrier.[12]

Revise your knowledge of current disability discrimination law and guidance appropriate to the locality in which you work, particularly that which covers training and development.

PASTORAL CARE

Learners will come to you with their own personalities and dispositions, their hopes and aspirations, past experiences and backgrounds, worries, responsibilities and anxieties. Very often it is inappropriate or unnecessary to enquire about these factors, but some teaching relationships can be affected by such 'external' factors, and they can obstruct learning.

The special context of healthcare teaching, dealing as it does with factors that influence health, life and death, has the potential to be especially challenging for learners. They may have to learn to deal with the sights, smells and sounds of pain, disease and death, difficult situations such as disturbed or abusive patients, variations in socioeconomic background of patients, and health inequalities that frustrate and surprise them. Some might be embarrassed or distressed about the discrepancy between their relative affluence and the circumstances of some patients. They may experience situations that mimic painful times in their own life, such as the death of a parent or child.

Learners are working in a sensitive environment where mistakes can have overwhelming consequences. They must learn to take responsibility for their decisions and take measured risks without being foolhardy or paralysed by fear of the consequences.

The role of the learner in a healthcare setting can be uncomfortable for these and many other reasons, and at the same time their behaviour and performance are under constant surveillance for what they show about their competence and their character.

Stress and anxiety will be heightened when members of staff are unfriendly or unsupportive and do not make learners feel welcome. Therefore it is important to control anxiety to a manageable level, recognise learners as beginners, acknowledge their insecurities and be aware that background factors may be affecting performance (*see* Box 18.5).

BOX 18.5 Providing support and supervision[13]

- Ensure that students feel able to seek help without loss of confidence or self-esteem, by attending to the way in which questions are answered and requests for support are handled.
- Foster self-confidence with praise and constructive feedback.
- Build in an element of choice about cases to which learners are exposed.
- Encourage self-monitoring and evaluation of performance.
- Give learners time to reflect on what has happened and what is happening, and promote discussion about patient care.
- Allow learners to make mistakes, but be aware of your power to manipulate events to allow success.

Space and time to reflect on traumatic cases and the role that the learner played are vital, both in terms of lessons to be learned and in terms of maintaining the health and well-being of trainees.

As healthcare providers you are used to caring and problem-solving roles, but there is a tension between these and your teaching role. Make sure that your learners are registered with a GP (outside your practice for those training in primary care), and do not provide personal healthcare advice. Be aware of, and appropriately signpost the way to, occupational health services, counsellors, relationship services, Citizens Advice Centres, the university or hospital chaplain, or other sources of advice and support.

Tips from experienced teachers

- Be aware of the power of role modelling as a way to reinforce desired behaviours.
- Be prepared to listen to and learn from the experiences that learners describe.
- Always allow time to debrief following significant events.
- Show confidence in the abilities of your learners; reinforce the expectation of success.

REFERENCES

1 Standing Committee on Postgraduate Medical and Dental Education. *An Enquiry into Mentoring: supporting doctors and dentists at work.* London: Standing Committee on Postgraduate Medical and Dental Education; 1998.

2 Duckitt K. Mentoring. *Women in Medicine Newsletter.* London: Women in Medicine; 1997.

3 Sandars J. Mentoring and peer-supported learning. *Update.* 1998; **November:** 760–1.

4 West Midlands Regional GP Education Committee. *Coaching and Mentoring Package.* Birmingham: West Midlands NHS Executive, GP Unit; 1995.

5 Lingam S, Gupta R. Mentoring for overseas doctors. Career focus. *BMJ.* 1998; **317:** 2–3.

6 Hamilton R. *Mentoring: a practical guide to the skills of mentoring.* London: Industrial Society; 1995.

7 Department of Postgraduate Medical and Dental Education, South and West. *Education Supervision: a handbook for hospital-based educational support.* PGMDE, South and West; 1997.

8 Sachdeva AK. Preceptorship, mentorship and the adult learner in medical and health sciences education. *J Cancer Educ.* 1996; **11:** 131–6.

9 Brown R, Hawksley B. *Learning Style, Studying Styles and Profiling.* London: Mark Allen Publishing; 1996.

10 Boyden T. Coaching for success. *Choices Newsletter.* Bristol: Executive Choice, NHS Senior Career Development Service, Dearden Management; 1999.

11 Rowntree D. *Assessing Students: how shall we know them?* 2nd edn. London: Kogan Page; 1987.

12 Halstead JA. Teaching students with special needs. In: Billings DM, Halstead JA, eds. *Teaching in Nursing: a guide for faculty.* Philadelphia, PA: WB Saunders; 1998.

13 Stuart C. *Assessment, Supervision and Support in Clinical Practice: a guide for nurses, midwives and other health professionals.* Edinburgh: Churchill Livingstone; 2003.

FURTHER READING

- *BMJ* Career Focus series: www.bmj.com
- Chambers R, Mohanna K, Field S. *Opportunities and Options in Medical Careers.* Oxford: Radcliffe Medical Press; 2000.
- Ward C, Eccles S. *So You Want To Be A Brain Surgeon? A medical careers guide.* 2nd edn. Oxford: Oxford Medical Publications; 2001.
- Wilson FC. Mentoring young physicians. In: *Graduate Medical Education.* Oxford: Radcliffe Publishing; 2009. pp. 93–8.

CHAPTER 19

Leadership training

Clinical engagement in leadership in healthcare is a key facet of professionalism. Leadership can be a difficult concept to recognise and develop in yourself and in your learners. However, all stages of the profession are looking to healthcare teachers for guidance and inspiration. Students might be in networks or looking for role models, juniors seek training opportunities and colleagues require ways to engage with and direct the future course of healthcare services. Healthcare professionals and managers must learn together to ensure integration and improved understanding of each others' roles. All of this requires innovative and exciting educational programmes. In the UK healthcare service, 'Leadership at all the levels' implies a diffused, situational leadership model. This chapter highlights the knowledge, skills and behaviours of effective clinical leaders, and explains how to spot, nurture and develop leadership potential in yourself and your learners.

Most recent thinking on healthcare leadership has concerned clinicians. Although there is considerable overlap in roles and responsibilities in healthcare these days, a need for greater medical engagement has been identified in two major reviews of UK healthcare organisation and provision.

'Talent management' in the healthcare service considers leadership as an integrated process rather than depending on individuals from a single profession, or being related to personality or personal traits. The responsibility for healthcare leadership rests with the most appropriate person (or team) at that particular time.

BACKGROUND

For UK doctors, an early call to leadership was made:

> The doctor's frequent role as head of the healthcare team and commander of considerable clinical resource requires that greater attention is paid to management and leadership skills regardless of specialism. An acknowledgement of the leadership role of medicine is increasingly evident.[1]

A controversial reform of UK postgraduate medical education and training under the policy initiative, Modernising Medical Careers, was aimed at speeding up the production of fully trained specialists. The speed with which these changes were introduced, coupled with an inadequate online application process supporting the first phase of change, resulted in widespread system deficiencies and countless tales of personal difficulties in career progression. The subsequent inquiry attributed fault to a policy that aspired to being 'good enough' rather than 'excellence' in training.[1] Aspiring to excellence would require doctors in particular, but also all others engaged in education and training, to step up as leaders in their profession.

The same inquiry identified confused or deficient professional engagement, particularly with regard to matters of education and training. As a result, a call was made for a lead for medical education, and stronger collaborations, particularly within the health education sector.[1] Suggestions for the integration of workforce policy objectives with training and service objectives, requiring a revision of the medical workforce planning process and increased external scrutiny, were also made. The medical profession has been urged to develop a mechanism for providing coherent advice on matters that affect the entire profession.

These recommendations require expansion of the number of healthcare professionals who are involved in aspects of leadership, and new training initiatives to equip them for this task. Furthermore, modifications are required for the structure of postgraduate training to provide a broad-based platform for subsequent higher specialist training, increased flexibility, the valuing of experience and the promotion of excellence.

A 2008 review of the UK NHS[2] placed emphasis on enabling healthcare staff to lead and manage the organisations in which they work:

> Greater freedom, enhanced accountability and empowering staff are necessary but not sufficient in the pursuit of high quality care. Making change actually happen takes leadership. It is central to our expectations of the healthcare professionals of tomorrow.[2]

In a move designed to 'enhance professionalism', suggestions have been made for investing in programmes of clinical and board leadership, with clinicians encouraged to be practitioners, partners and leaders in the healthcare system. In the UK, a National Leadership Council (NLC) was suggested to create a step change in the development of leadership, 'responsible for overseeing all matters of leadership across healthcare'.[2] The consultation process that informed the NLC development emphasised that the drive for leadership should permeate all levels and grades of the healthcare organisation. There is a strong emphasis on clinical leadership, but a similar drive for the NLC to work with people and professional groups from all backgrounds.

The identification and development of leadership potential have four underpinning principles:[3]

1 co-production – the engagement of people across 'the system' to work together to make change happen
2 subsidiarity – ensuring that decisions are made at the right level, and as close to the user as possible
3 clinical ownership and leadership – building on the concept of staff as 'practitioners, partners and leaders'
4 system alignment – aligning different parts of the system towards the same goals as a way of achieving complex cultural change.

The NHS is now seeking medical engagement to help to address efficiencies in the NHS through the Quality, Innovation, Productivity and Prevention (QIPP) agenda, and in this context, leadership development.

DEVELOPING LEADERSHIP POTENTIAL IN OTHERS

How can you help to develop leadership potential in others? Many different and varied theories of leadership (and management) make even an overview confusing.[4] The three categories of leadership approach are as follows (further details can be found in other sources[4,5]):

➤ trait theory: emphasises personal qualities
➤ situational leadership: suggests that different tasks call for different leaders with a varying skill mix
➤ transactional or transformational leadership: transactional leadership relying on incentives and exchanges to engender followership, and transformational leadership depending more on the empowering of individuals.

It is most useful to consider what leaders do, rather than what their qualities are. A UK project, 'Enhancing Medical Engagement', addressed the precise 'managerial' and 'leadership' roles that healthcare organisations seek from clinicians. To widen clinicians' involvement in leadership roles and leadership development, the National Institute for Innovation and Improvement (www.institute.nhs.uk) developed two leadership qualities frameworks (www.NHSLeadershipQualities.nhs.uk). One of these, the National Leadership Qualities Framework, lists behaviours under the following three themes:

➤ personal characteristics
➤ setting direction
➤ delivering the service.

This is an aspirational framework for established practitioners to develop as clinical or medical directors. The Medical Leadership Competency Framework applies to medical students and doctors, recognising that leadership is an integral part of the position. Depending on the stage of the professional's career, a differential range of competences is expected within each category.

TEACHING AND LEARNING ACTIVITIES

Multiple teaching and learning activities can help you to develop leaders among your learners.

Multisource feedback (MSF, or 360 degree assessment)

An effective conduit for development as professionals, team members and leaders is through eliciting and responding to feedback. A 360 degree assessment tool, developed by the NHS Institute for Innovation and Improvement, seeks to assess how team members view the behaviours of a potential leader. Thus it identifies areas to be developed or particular strengths of an individual.

Shadowing

Buddying potential leaders with colleagues in positions of influence in other organisations can allow 'cross-fertilisation' of ideas, close observation at first hand and the development of transferable qualities. By occasionally spending time in another's workplace, you can compare and contrast the qualities and behaviours that are required for success.

Experimentation or simulation

Leadership development programmes often include simulation exercises. This provides a safe environment in which variables can be adjusted to test out actions and reactions in a team arena, with different individuals taking the position of leader. Both on courses and in the workplace, exercises can be developed for departments and teams to practise acting under pressure.

ADDIE (Analysis, Design, Develop, Implement, Evaluate)[6]

ADDIE refers to a system that was originally developed for instructional media design (primarily in e-learning), which can be adapted to become a form of project development exercise. This can be used as the basis of an effective game for thinking about leadership activity (*see* Box 19.1).

BOX 19.1 The ADDIE game (Analyse, Design, Develop, Implement, Evaluate)

This is an exercise for two small mixed-professional groups.

Preamble: Swine flu has hit the hospital, and 20 temporary staff at all levels have been brought in to help with the peak season.
Task: Design a short activity that will allow the permanent employees to meet and introduce themselves to the temporary staff and decide who will do what during the emergency season.

Analyse the problem: Perform a short task analysis. How do people usually get to know each other?
Design the activity: Develop objectives, sequence.
Develop the activity: Outline how they will perform the activity and trial it.
Implement the activity: Describe the activity to the other group.
Evaluate the activity: Groups vote on both schemes.

Organisational support

Leaders do not emerge overnight. Leadership capacity must be proactively developed within an organisation to encourage new leaders. Some organisations are better at this than others. Effective organisations encourage mentoring in the workplace (*see* Chapter 18). Box 19.2[4] shows how effective organisations support and encourage new leadership.

> **BOX 19.2** Organisational support for developing leaders (modified from Cragg, in Chambers and Mohanna *et al.*[4])
>
> An effective mentor should ensure that inexperienced leaders set realistic and challenging objectives while enabling effective use of the fresh perspective and energy that they bring. Achievable goals with a degree of responsibility and influence promote personal development and motivation. Effective interim evaluation, during as well as after the project, should assess the success of developmental opportunities and give essential feedback to the learner. Ensure that you develop training and development opportunities for those in existing positions of leadership, as well as for inexperienced newcomers.

Practice-based learning

With a supportive organisation, aspiring leaders can experiment in the higher-stakes setting of a practice-based project. Leaders must have innovative ideas and the ability to implement change. A project that is under their control but effectively supervised will unearth hidden abilities. To minimise the risk that funding will disappear part of the way through, as priorities change, you should ensure that there is active engagement by the organisation so that projects can be discussed and developed together with the aspiring leader, and that activities are as congruent with the development plan of the organisation as they are with that of the project lead.

CONCLUSION: LEADERSHIP AND CREATIVITY

There is much interest in the way in which 'creativity' might apply to healthcare service development. Effective leaders frequently provide new direction, inspiration and ideas, which implies imagination and creativity. However, if their function is to be catalysts, their main roles may be to recognise or enable creativity in others.

Perhaps creative leaders are those who can find better ways of doing things, either themselves or through others. However, if such inspiration is associated with inadequate communication skills, this situated leadership (leadership demonstrated at the point where it is needed) might go unnoticed. To ensure implementation, creative leadership must be associated with 'followership.'

Be aware of the oscillating position of individuals, who may sometimes be leaders and at other times followers. Mutual respect, open-mindedness and the ability to speak up and to listen are essential leadership qualities.

Aspiring leaders might become disillusioned about the ability of the healthcare system to react and respond to challenge. You can protect learners from the risks of cynicism by helping them to develop as 'imaginative professionals.'[6,7] This model links the inner world of values with the external world of public policy, and predicts that some protection can be obtained against the corrosive effects of 'performativity.' This process aspires to raise standards by looking directly at outcomes, rather than inputs or processes. It can infuriate healthcare professionals who characterise it as a 'tick-box' exercise. Healthcare leadership needs to find a new voice. By engaging with the process of change in healthcare through leadership and speaking out about the shared values of healthcare workers, you can cultivate an environment in which 'creative professionalism', a new inclusive discourse, can flourish.[8]

Examples of established training programmes

➤ **The King's Fund:** 'Developing confident, able and imaginative leaders within the NHS for more than 30 years' (www.kingsfund.org.uk/leadership/index.html).

➤ **National Health Service:** NHS Graduate Management Training Scheme, the Gateway to Leadership Programme ('for experienced employees from other industries') or the Breaking Through Programme ('seeking to develop successful leaders from black and minority ethnic backgrounds') (www.nhsleadtheway. co.uk).

➤ **Royal College of Nursing (RCN) Clinical Leadership Programme:** This programme can be commissioned by an organisation which nominates a lead to attend an RCN facilitators' programme and run the programme on site within their organisation (www.rcn.org.uk/development/practice/leadership).

➤ **Royal College of General Practitioners:** 'give general practice a voice in shaping the future of UK healthcare' (www.rcgp.org.uk/professional_development/ leadership_programme.aspx).

➤ **Association for the Study of Medical Education:** 'to allow participants to deliver professional, organisational objectives in healthcare education' (www. asme.org.uk).

REFERENCES

1 Tooke J. *Aspiring to Excellence: findings and final recommendations of the Independent Inquiry into Modernising Medical Careers.* London: MMC Inquiry; 2008. www.mmcinquiry.org.uk/ Final_8_Jan_08_MMC_all.pdf

2 Darzi A. *High Quality Care for All. NHS next stage review.* London: Department of Health; 2008. www.dh.gov.uk/prod_consum_dh/groups/dh_digitalassets/@dh/@en/ documents/digitalasset/dh_085828.pdf

3 Department of Health Workforce Directorate. *Inspiring Leaders: leadership for quality.* London: Department of Health; 2009. www.dh.gov.uk/prod_consum_dh/groups/ dh_digitalassets/documents/digitalasset/dh_093407.pdf

4 Chambers R, Mohanna K, Spurgeon P. *How to Succeed as a Leader.* Oxford: Radcliffe Publishing; 2007.

5 Wilkie V, Spurgeon P. *Management for New GPs.* London: Royal College of General Practitioners; 2009.

6 Allen M. *Creating Successful e-Learning: a rapid system for getting it right first time, every time.* San Francisco, CA: Pfeiffer; 2006.

7 Power S. The imaginative professional. In: Cunningham B, ed. *Exploring Professionalism.* London: Institute of Education; 2008.

8 Barnett R. Critical professionalism in an age of supercomplexity. In: Cunningham B, ed. *Exploring Professionalism.* London: Institute of Education; 2008.

CHAPTER 20

Applying education and training to the requirements of the healthcare system

In the past, teachers taught subjects in isolation, without considering the relevance or consequences of that teaching on the whole healthcare system or on different disciplines. Teachers may have focused on improving practice in one topic regardless of whether it was a priority for the healthcare system or learner. Teaching about one topic without alluding to the knock-on effects, such as the consequent lack of resources for other areas of practice, or setting a poor role model by not considering the perspectives of patients or those in other disciplines, might be considered irresponsible.

This chapter considers ideas for teaching some of the challenging areas of practice, including the following:
➤ clinical governance
➤ involving the public and patients in the planning and delivery of healthcare
➤ putting changes into practice
➤ involving patients in teaching.

Many of these skills require the development of the organisation as well as teaching individual professionals specific skills. Leaders of clinical governance must learn how to motivate others while taking a wider perspective that encompasses the work of other management and clinical professionals. Individual practitioners should link their clinical practice closely with research evidence, and must listen to the views of patients and the public with regard to healthcare system priorities.

TEACHING ABOUT CLINICAL GOVERNANCE

Clinical governance is about implementing care within an environment in which clinical effectiveness can flourish, by establishing a facilitatory culture. Implementation of clinical governance is only possible if practitioners know what it is (*see* Box 20.1), what the organisation requires, and how to apply appropriate knowledge, skills and attitudes in practice. Education in isolation from active practice or without the necessary resources (e.g. skills, access to information technology, and the time available to professionals and non-clinical staff to undertake the associated work) cannot achieve the successful implementation of clinical governance.

BOX 20.1 Components of clinical governance
(adapted from the National Centre for Clinical Audit[1])

- Clinical audit.
- Risk management.
- Evidence-based clinical practice.
- Development of clinical leadership skills.
- Managing the clinical performance of colleagues.
- Continuing education/professional development for all staff.
- Health needs assessment.
- Learning from mistakes.
- Effective management of poorly performing colleagues.

Teaching about the meaning of clinical governance

Clinical governance cannot be taught effectively from the perspective of a single discipline in a classroom, because establishing clinical governance necessitates a change in culture. Teaching should address knowledge, skills and attitudes, as well as more complex learning, such as that about negotiation, political awareness and finding out others' opinions, roles and responsibilities. Effective implementation of clinical governance requires the whole organisation to be flexible to change in response to individuals' learning and application of clinical governance in their workplaces.

A combination of activities, such as paper-based and electronic newsletters, workshops, lectures, seminars and tutorials, could deliver education about the meaning of clinical governance. The components of clinical governance were originally set out in a UK government White Paper.[2] Since then, different organisations[1,3,4] have applied the meaning of clinical governance to their special areas of interest (*see* Boxes 20.1–20.5). Learners could compile a portfolio describing their contribution to their practice's or unit's programme of developments or overall clinical governance effort.

BOX 20.2 Approach adopted by the Royal College of
General Practitioners[3] to clinical governance

Protecting patients
- Registration/revalidation of professional qualifications.
- Identifying unacceptable variations in care and areas in need of improvement.
- Managing and minimising poor performance of colleagues.
- Risk management.

Developing people
- Continuing professional development or lifelong learning.
- Development and implementation of guidelines and protocols for 'best practice.'
- Personal accreditation.
- Recognising and celebrating success.

Developing teams and systems
- Learning from what other teams do well.

- Clinical audit.
- Development and implementation of guidelines and protocols for 'best practice'.
- Recognising and celebrating success.
- Evidence-based clinical practice.
- Improving cost-effectiveness.
- Listening to the views of patients and carers.
- Practice accreditation.
- Through all of the above, promoting accountability and transparency.

A baseline for individual learners might be as follows:
- to identify their own learning needs and plan an appropriate educational programme
- to know something of their organisation's strategic or business plan
- to have basic skills in critical appraisal and searching for evidence relevant to best practice in their field
- to know the government's clinical priorities relating to them
- to be able to undertake clinical audit
- to know what constitutes clinical and non-clinical risks in the course of their work or in the workplace
- to understand accountability and its relationship to the healthcare system
- to be engaged in risk minimisation and know how to act if a significant event occurs
- to know how to involve consumers and act on their feedback as an integral part of day-to-day work.

BOX 20.3 Processes for clinical governance adopted by the Royal College of Nursing[4]

- Patient- or client-focused approach.
- Integrated approach to managing and improving quality.
- Effective multi-professional teamwork.
- Information sharing and networking.
- Open culture: learning from mistakes.

When teaching learners about the implementation of clinical governance, you are likely to encounter the following challenges.
➤ Teaching the theory when the infrastructure and resources (information technology and software, data collection, support and accountability systems) practising in this way are inadequate.
➤ The managers and chief executives of healthcare organisations possibly having little understanding of the topic and how to facilitate its application.
➤ Teaching evidence-based practice to individuals whose colleagues do little to follow suit.
➤ Encouraging professionals to own standards or guidelines of good practice, or to set their own.
➤ Running multi-professional CPD[5] when professionals from single disciplines cling to their territorial traditions.

➤ Teaching about national priorities and establishing the extent and nature of their local adoption where there may be conflicting guidelines.
➤ Limited knowledge of the evidence for and constraints on best practice in prescribing.
➤ Teaching professionals to view 'health' as a broad concept that encompasses physical, mental, social and environmental well-being.
➤ Teaching the benefits of a learning, non-blaming culture when professionals operate in a competitive environment, and mistakes and complaints are viewed as serious failures.
➤ Teaching the theory of cost-effectiveness when there are few systems for fair and responsible prioritisation of resources at local or national levels.
➤ Learning how to establish meaningful user/non-user involvement in policy, planning and monitoring of care.
➤ Understanding the legal implications of containment of demand and maintenance of performance standards.
➤ Motivating learners to want to make change work when multiple ongoing amendments to healthcare system policies and priorities have left them 'change fatigued.'
➤ Finding protected time to do the work involved in undertaking clinical governance effectively.

Promoting understanding about what the organisation requires will focus on making sure that the principles of good practice in the application of clinical governance are fulfilled in a coordinated way across the patch. These will include:
➤ delivering local priorities such as those in the healthcare organisation's local delivery plan
➤ addressing national healthcare priorities
➤ clinical and management practices being based on best evidence as far as possible
➤ setting up structures and systems for delivering the components of clinical governance.

Teaching the application of clinical governance in practice will require education about how to:
➤ establish and maintain a quality improvement culture
➤ motivate others to integrate the core components of clinical governance into their everyday work
➤ evaluate changes in practice
➤ specify and measure health gains
➤ use the most appropriate type of consumer involvement for particular settings or situations
➤ obtain and apply information about populations or clinical matters.

Your clinical governance educational programme might have a multi-pronged approach, as follows:
➤ Teaching practitioners different ways to find out about patients' concerns and what they would like to see changed (the term 'patient' is used here to include user, non-user, carer and the general public).[6]

➤ Teaching managers how to organise a coherent plan for clinical governance across their practice, unit or organisation. This will involve knowing what the priorities are in relation to the organisation's strategic goals, and may include any and every aspect of organisational development, mapping out baseline resources, undertaking a needs assessment, improving information systems and establishing a learning, non-blaming culture.

➤ Teaching clinicians how to identify and agree several priorities on which to focus their clinical governance development in accordance with both the organisation's priorities and their own professional priorities.

➤ Teaching non-clinical staff to identify and agree several priorities for clinical governance in line with the priorities of both the organisation and their clinical colleagues. Ensuring that those in supportive posts realise that their contribution is vital for healthcare professionals to be able to provide effective face-to-face care.

➤ Encouraging each set of staff as uni-disciplinary or multi-professional groups to develop action plans in those agreed priority areas that either incorporate the core components or justify why core components are not relevant. Their action plans should make the purpose, process, expected outcomes and people's roles and responsibilities clear.

➤ Encouraging interaction between managers and healthcare professions should ensure that the 'bottom-up' priorities are consistent with 'top-down' priorities. This should help managers to see that healthcare professionals have the resources necessary to implement clinical governance, and healthcare professionals to view managers in a positive light with regard to improvement in the quality of care and services.

➤ Teaching those involved in implementing clinical governance the importance of monitoring progress and outcomes and revising associated action programmes as necessary.

➤ Developing a learning culture within the organisation, and developing new ways of working and problem solving.[7]

TEACHING INVOLVEMENT OF THE PUBLIC AND PATIENTS IN THE PLANNING AND DELIVERY OF HEALTHCARE

It is difficult to teach the theory of involving the public and patients in the planning or delivery of healthcare without learners also obtaining first-hand practical experience. When required to establish what people think, many health professionals turn to a questionnaire survey. This has many disadvantages – for example, the great potential for exclusion of elderly, visually impaired, mentally ill and homeless people, depending on how participants are identified and the actual method that is chosen. Teachers must therefore have considerable practical knowledge and understanding of ways in which biases in sampling and processing surveys can be minimised.[6,8]

Such teaching requires a combination of knowledge and application of research methodology, information gathering, management, health policy, needs assessments, health economics and communication (*see* Box 20.4). Some teaching may be delivered through traditional methods such as lectures, seminars and workshops describing others' experiences. However, you must also provide opportunities for facilitated hands-on experience, perhaps by:

➤ linking a less experienced practice or unit with ones that have undertaken successful consultation exercises previously
➤ inviting an expert facilitator to lead a group of professionals through the planning and execution of real examples
➤ arranging 'shadowing' to allow less experienced professionals to observe more expert professionals undertaking a planned consultation.

BOX 20.4 Criteria that should be taught as good practice in any exercise that involves and engages the public or patients in the planning or delivery of healthcare[8]

- Specify the purpose of the consultation.
- Create a timetabled programme at the planning stage. Include details of the aim, method, expected outcomes, feedback and review.
- Ensure that the method of obtaining the views of users, carers and the public is appropriate for the question posed and the information required.
- The exercise should be necessary. Is the information already available elsewhere?
- Select an appropriate method and be able to justify this choice.
- There should be sufficient resources to carry out a well-constructed consultation process.
- Lay involvement should be sought and achieved at an early stage in the process of planning or providing care.
- Seek statistical advice early on to find out how many people to survey and check the design.
- Feed back the results to those who contributed to the exercise.
- Decisions or changes should be made as a result of the exercise. If they were not, this lack of change should be justified.
- The consultation process should involve a representative group of people central to the purpose of the consultation. The extent to which the target population groups were included, the processes by which the citizens were involved, the response rates and whether the consultation process favoured representatives with particular skills should all be stated.
- The learner should be aware of the impacts, benefits and drawbacks of involvement of the public.
- The learner should be aware of how conflicts of interest (e.g. competing priorities) were resolved.

INVOLVING PATIENTS IN TEACHING

Consider training patients to become effective teachers, or involving them in teaching healthcare teachers about utilising patients as teachers.

Patients can be trained to become standardised patients – that is, patients who have a specific condition and are taught to present themselves consistently to allow healthcare students or professionals to practise, or be assessed on, communication, diagnostic or examination skills. Standardised patients are not to be confused with simulated patients. The latter are actors who are trained to present themselves as having a particular condition. The consistency fostered by using either standardised or simulated patients is beneficial for the purposes of assessment. Learners are able to test different management approaches in a 'safe' environment, and to obtain feedback about the effectiveness of each – a unique and invaluable opportunity that cannot be provided in the clinical setting.

In order to develop patients as effective teachers, you must teach them to succeed when faced with presentations, meetings, focus groups, surveys, role playing and facilitation. When considering utilising patients as teachers, you should address the following issues:

➤ commitment, building trust, and engaging with, empowering and promoting the inclusion of patients as teachers
➤ practical issues (e.g. travel, parking, accessibility, communication)
➤ respecting patients and taking their diverse and individual needs into account
➤ being open to a variety of user-led materials (e.g. calendars, photographs, poetry, art, video and theatre)
➤ prompt and appropriate payment and non-monetary rewards
➤ power and empowering patients.

BOX 20.5 Key components of patient-centred care for which it could be particularly beneficial to involve patients as teachers

- Partnership: help for someone with a problem, achieved through partnership between that person and health professionals.
- Empowerment: help for patients with problems to find the best ways of helping themselves.
- Judgement: the person with the problem is the only one who really understands their experience and problem.
- Values: people's values and priorities change with time. They may be quite different from the health professional's values, but no less valid.
- Autonomy: a fundamental right of every individual. Illness, disability, low income, unemployment and other forms of social exclusion mean a loss of some aspects of autonomy in society.
- Listening: active non-judgemental listening is core to helping people, and crucial to gaining an understanding of people's problems.
- Shared decision making: people with ongoing problems need to be able to take their own decisions about the care of their clinical condition, based on expert information communicated to them by health professionals. Patients do value shared decision making, but not as much as other key attributes of consultations, such as having a doctor or nurse who listens, and being provided with easily understood information. Shared decision making leads to concordance, which should be the goal of all shared decision-making encounters between health professional and patient.

Focus on helping learners to appreciate what patient-centred healthcare delivery means (*see* Box 20.5), and the balance to be achieved between patients' needs and preferences. Patients in a teaching role will have more impact on learners than a professional teacher when discussing the feelings of vulnerability, isolation and loss of control that accompany illness. Patient-teachers can help learners to appreciate the potential power imbalance that is created by the superior knowledge of the healthcare professional. They can promote shared decision making as the middle ground between informed choice, where decisions are left entirely to the patient, and traditional, paternalistic medical decision making. This means two-way information giving (medical and personal) between the clinician and the patient concerning all of the options available, with the final decision being made jointly.

Tips from experienced teachers

If you do recruit patients as teachers of health professionals and/or managers, prepare them well and look after them.

- Be clear about the purpose.
- Target the patient contribution for maximum gain. Don't exhaust them or keep them hanging around.
- Enable your patient-teacher to be well prepared and confident. Describe the nature of the learners and what sort of things will be most useful for them to hear about.
- Protect the patient from the 'audience'. Don't allow the patient-teacher to be hassled or to be expected to answer questions that are too challenging or personal.
- Encourage learners to realise the benefits of hearing the patient's perspective at first hand.

TEACHING ABOUT CHANGE

Much is known about the effects of change on an organisation and workforce. However, the gaps between theory and practice[9] and the general lack of application of research into clinical practice are well recognised. This is the focus of translational medicine. Effective ways of teaching about changing practice, such that those changes are widely put into place, continue to be elusive.

People underestimate the barriers and hurdles to be overcome before change will be made and sustained. These barriers include the following:[10]

➤ lack of perception of relevance
➤ lack of resources
➤ short-term outlook
➤ conflicting priorities
➤ difficulty in measuring outcomes
➤ lack of necessary skills
➤ no history of multi-disciplinary working
➤ limitations of the research evidence on effectiveness
➤ perverse incentives
➤ intensity of contribution required.

Any teaching programme that is intended to involve and motivate learners to effect changes in practice must address the barriers that the individual learner can influence. It should also provide the necessary additional knowledge and skills for learners to be able to understand the need for change and the practical means to put change into practice. Even then, change will not be possible unless healthcare service managers are committed to it and are prepared to alter the environment to make it happen.

You must help learners to understand how people react to change (*see* Figure 20.1). Initially they are surprised, even if change is anticipated. Then they move from surprise/ shock to denying that it will happen.[11]

After the denial phase they look for somebody to blame for what has happened

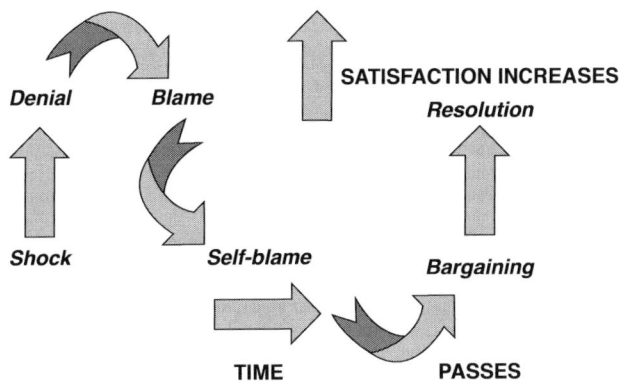

FIGURE 20.1

– often the individual(s) who announce the change. After general blame comes self-blame.

Part of the next stage, the bargaining, involves negotiating that if they do it *this* way they are going to be able to do *that*. Eventually they arrive at the resolution phase, where they have accepted the organisational change.

Different people pass through the stages of change differently according to individual and situational factors. When change is imposed, people are generally much more resistant and move more slowly. If the effect of the change is serious, feelings about it will be stronger and longer will be spent in the denial, blame and self-blame stages.

Planning for change

You must teach learners to address change by clarifying where they are heading and identifying the causes of dissatisfaction. Learners should plan how to reach their target and find their way in staged steps to measure their progress.

Learners should be taught to recognise the roles that people play in response to change. For example:
➤ the rebel – 'I don't see why I should'
➤ the victim – 'I suppose you will make me, but I will drag my feet'
➤ the oppressor – 'You all have to do it'
➤ the rescuer – 'I will save you all from this terrible change.'

Tips for making changes

Give learners a checklist for planning change that they can adapt to their particular situation.
➤ Have realistic time scales and be flexible.
➤ Provide clear communication about what is happening.
➤ Consult with all staff, identifying all problems as they occur.
➤ Plan for more resources and time than you expect to use.
➤ Fix interval markers of progress.
➤ Feed information back to everyone about what is happening.
➤ Identify anxieties and try to resolve them.

➤ Consider the effects of this change on other services and people.
➤ Beware of too many changes taking place at once.
➤ Recognise that change can be hijacked by vested interests, and the direction altered.
➤ Be prepared to change direction if necessary.
➤ Beware of a lack of commitment from others.

Motivating people to change, to do a better job

The best way to discover what motivates people is to ask them. People are motivated by different things. Some of the best motivators for fulfilling health professionals' needs are:
➤ interesting and/or useful work
➤ a sense of achievement
➤ responsibility
➤ opportunities for career progression or professional development
➤ gaining new skills or competences
➤ a sense of belonging to a healthcare organisation or practice team
➤ personal or written congratulations from a respected colleague or immediate superior
➤ public recognition
➤ announcement of success at team meetings
➤ recognising that the last job was well done and asking for an opinion on the next one
➤ providing specific and frequent feedback (positive feedback first)
➤ providing information on how the task has affected the performance of the organisation or the management of a patient
➤ encouragement to increase their knowledge and skills to do even better
➤ making time to listen to ideas, complaints or difficulties
➤ learning from mistakes and making visible changes.

Human nature makes people respond better to praise than to punishment. So when you teach others about motivation, emphasise the importance of praise and celebrating people's achievements.

As with any feedback, start with the positive things (*see* Chapter 13). Praise should come:
➤ immediately after the successful completion of part or all of a particular task
➤ from someone who knows what the task involved (not a remote committee)
➤ from an understanding of what the task involved.

REFERENCES

1 National Centre for Clinical Audit. *Autumn Newsletter*. London: National Centre for Clinical Audit; 1998.
2 National Health Service Executive. *The New NHS: modern, dependable*. London: Department of Health; 1997.
3 Royal College of General Practitioners. *Practical Advice on the Implementation of Clinical Governance in Primary Care in England and Wales*. London: Royal College of General Practitioners; 1999.

4 Royal College of Nursing. *Guidance for Nurses on Clinical Governance.* London: Royal College of Nursing; 1998.

5 Standing Committee on Postgraduate Medical and Dental Education. *Multi-Professional Working and Learning: sharing the educational challenge.* London: Standing Committee on Postgraduate Medical and Dental Education; 1997.

6 McIver S. *Obtaining the Views of Health Service Users about Quality of Information.* London: King's Fund; 1993.

7 Garcarz W, Chambers R, Ellis S. *Make Your Healthcare Organisation a Learning Organisation.* Oxford: Radcliffe Medical Press; 2003.

8 Chambers R, Drinkwater C, Boath E. *Involving Patients and the Public.* 2nd edn. Oxford: Radcliffe Medical Press; 2003.

9 Chief Nursing Officer. *Integrating Theory and Practice in Nursing.* Leeds: NHS Executive; 1998.

10 Dunning M, Abi-Aad G, Gilbert D *et al. Turning Evidence into Everyday Practice.* London: King's Fund; 1998.

11 Chambers R, Wakley G, Iqbal Z *et al. Prescription for Learning: techniques, games and activities.* Oxford: Radcliffe Medical Press; 2002.

FURTHER READING

• Association of Standardized Patient Educators: www.aspeducators.org/sp_info.htm
• Chambers R, Wakley G, Iqbal Z *et al.* Managing change. In: *Prescription for Learning: techniques, games and activities.* Oxford: Radcliffe Medical Press; 2002.
• INVOLVE: www.invo.org.uk

CHAPTER 21

Best-evidence medical education

Best-evidence medical education is as important as any other evidence-based aspect of healthcare, and has been defined as:

> the implementation, by teachers in their practice, of methods and approaches to education based on the best evidence available.[1]

This chapter introduces the underlying concepts of best-evidence medical education, highlights the difficulties with this, suggests a pragmatic approach to practising in this way, and provides information on adding to the evidence by undertaking medical education research.

EVIDENCE-BASED EDUCATION

Increasingly people are asking for evidence of what does and what does not work in medical education, along the lines of evidence-based medicine.[2] There are signs that this is also happening in education in general. In 2000, the Secretary of State for Education for England suggested that:

> We need . . . social scientists to tell us what works and why and what types of policy initiatives are likely to be most effective. And we need better ways of ensuring that those who want the information can get it easily and quickly.[3]

His counterpart in Scotland also expressed his surprise at 'how little science there is done in education', and suggested that educational researchers should 'sharpen up on the scientific methods they use and . . . make sure they drop the value judgements within them.'[4]

This has produced a furious debate within the educational literature. Hargreaves supports this evidence-based approach and maintains that educational research should and could have more relevance and impact upon the professional practice of teachers than it does at present.[5] He outlines parallels between education and medicine, and the way medical research relates to professional practice. Opposition views are that no hard evidence exists of what works to help teachers to teach better, and that such evidence cannot be obtained in the field of education.[6] Another critic has questioned whether we should follow the evidence-based movement in education 'like lemmings.'[4]

However, arguments are not productive. You just want to know what does and what does not work in real life. Do learners learn as a result of your efforts, or in spite of them? Could you be making things worse? The answers to these questions may lie in the best-evidence medical education movement.

BEST-EVIDENCE MEDICAL EDUCATION

Healthcare professionals are trained to make clinical decisions that are based on evidence. However, when it comes to teaching, many abandon this approach and base everything on tradition and intuition – the PHOG method (prejudices, hunches, opinions and guesses).[7] When new ideas are introduced, very little real, reliable or valid evidence may be available, and these ideas may subsequently be found to be unhelpful and wasteful of time, effort and resources. Medical education may develop on the basis of fad and fashions, new ideas and new theories, with little or no evidence base.[8]

Even when evidence exists, integrating best-evidence medical education into teaching programmes may be problematic. For example, a randomised trial demonstrated the superiority of tapes/slides over lectures,[9] yet enthusiasm for lectures continues.

Healthcare teachers often believe that evidence to support or reject educational approaches is not available. Students of medical education often argue against principles of educational theory on the grounds that 'there is no evidence that they work.' This is sometimes true, but in other circumstances evidence is not found because it is sought in the wrong place, using inappropriate databases (e.g. Medline).

> There is a huge body of evidence out there but it is either not known about or ignored.[10]

The absence of enthusiasm for sufficient, rigorous academic inquiry and the implementation of existing positive evidence, together with the persistence of traditional methods, are limiting development.

Can we obtain substantive evidence for what we do? Randomised controlled trials (RCTs) in education are impractical and, perhaps, illogical.[11] Research design must be matched to the question, and an RCT may not be the gold standard in all cases. Even Sackett, the 'father' of evidence-based medicine, has now recanted his previous dogmatic support of the RCT, and suggests that attempting to choose a best overall design is an oversimplification.[12] Mixed methods can be used to research the effectiveness of educational interventions, just as they are used to evaluate new clinical treatments.

There are problems with funding this type of work. Directors of research and development appear to prefer the RCT design, so educational researchers sometimes struggle to convey their messages.

What do we need to do?

The six steps of evidence-based teaching can be summarised as follows:
1 framing the question
2 developing a search strategy

3 producing the raw data
4 evaluating the evidence
5 implementing change
6 evaluating that change.

Health professionals have limited time in which to search the literature, but a carefully planned 'search strategy' should result in quick identification of important publications. A good search strategy[13] will have a well-framed question relating to the purpose of the enquiry, and key words chosen specifically to reflect the dimensions of the question to use with appropriate databases. You must seek and grade the power of evidence to find out what works and what does not work. Critically appraise the literature to identify gaps, flaws and the need for further studies. Even if you are not involved in reviews or undertaking research, an understanding of the principles of best-evidence medical education is important if you are to implement it in your practice.

Seeking out the best evidence for medical education involves three key tasks:[14]

1 preparation of systematic reviews of suitable rigour and merit
2 dissemination of the results of this work
3 nurturing a culture of respect and value for medical teaching equal to that of other aspects of professional practice.

Just as with the Cochrane Collaboration, where evidence-based medicine, reviews of evidence and meta-analyses of various medical interventions are collated, the beginnings of a series of reviews in the areas of evidence-based teaching, and evidence-based policy and practice, are appearing in education. These systematic reviews are part of the Campbell Collaboration.

Best-evidence medical education: some examples

The evaluation of problem-based education within a Canadian and an Australian medical school is a good example of evidence-based medical education. These courses consist of some lectures and seminars, but also a lot of small group work, private study and personal tutorials. The evidence suggests that this results in improved student satisfaction, improved evaluations and better performance.[15]

Another example is a review of the teaching of communication skills,[16] which concluded that:

➤ communication skills can be taught
➤ they are learned
➤ communication skills are best maintained by practice
➤ teaching should be experiential, not instructional
➤ contents should be problem defining
➤ the least competent students improve the most
➤ men take longer to learn than women do.

Therefore good-quality evidence shows us that communication skills can be taught and learned, and there is good evidence to inform teachers on how best to teach them using experiential methods (patients, role players, video recording and constructive feedback on performance). However, educationalists are still frequently requested to give a lecture on communication skills.

Beware of the traps associated with gathering evidence on the effectiveness of teaching interventions. Consider another review which looked at the value of journal clubs in postgraduate medical education.[17] Here the authors searched 10 databases and found 63 studies on the subject. They used a rigorous Cochrane type of review for their inclusion criteria, and were left with only six studies on which to base their conclusions, which were that journal clubs may:

➤ improve knowledge of clinical epidemiology and statistics
➤ improve reading habits
➤ improve the use of medical literature in clinical practice.

They then called for a multicentre RCT to assess whether journal clubs worked! Presumably the doctors who were to be randomised to the control groups would attend journal clubs where no journals were discussed, or attend meetings where they did not realise a journal club was taking place, or attend an event and not even realise they were in a meeting at all!

Much does depend on how you review the evidence, and what you include and exclude.[18] In the future, hopefully, there will be further expert reviews on key topics in medical education.

CHALLENGES FOR EVIDENCE-BASED TEACHING

There are different levels of outcomes that you can evaluate when looking at your teaching (*see* Chapter 16). Referring to Kirkpatrick's hierarchy, many evaluation tools look at lower-order outcomes such as participants' reactions and changes in their knowledge base. The evidence base for teaching initiatives would be more powerful and clinically relevant if higher-order outcomes were evaluated. There are three main barriers to this:

1 the 'distance' between the input (the teaching strategy) and the output (the change in healthcare)
2 external factors such as learners' prior knowledge, motivation, opportunity, access to materials, time constraints, emotional and even financial pressures can affect learning
3 not all learning results from your teaching – some learning happens in spite of it. Well-motivated learners can overcome deficiencies in teaching.[19] If you use improvements in healthcare as a proxy marker for good healthcare teaching, you may be measuring the impact of factors that have nothing to do with your teaching.

> Compared to medicine, research in education may be more complex, confounding factors may be more apparent, content may be more implicit and controlled trials may be difficult.[8]

However, it is not impossible. A modified hierarchy of evaluation was used in a review of inter-professional education.[18] Based on the Kirkpatrick hierarchy, it has four levels and six categories:

➤ level 1: learners' reactions
➤ level 2a: modification of attitudes and perceptions
➤ level 2b: acquisition of knowledge and skills
➤ level 3: change in behaviour

➤ level 4a: change in organisational practice
➤ level 4b: benefits to patients/clients.

The top level in the hierarchy relates to benefits to patients as a direct result of the educational programme. It is possible to evaluate higher-order outcomes, but 'quick and dirty' research often fails to take these long-term outcomes into account. It may require the skills of epidemiologists and public health professionals to look at how aspects of your teaching affect the health of patients and populations.[18]
    Educational research can, and should, take many forms. Study designs could include:
➤ experimental studies
➤ observational studies
➤ case studies
➤ ethnographic studies
➤ experiential studies
➤ natural experiments.

However, this variety compounds the problems of evaluating evidence, as it is not always clear how to categorise the types of evidence that are being evaluated. A study in Birmingham highlighted this challenge.[20] Reviewers were paired off and asked to categorise various studies from the abstracts of published papers. Working independently, there was a surprisingly low degree of correlation between reviewers.

EDUCATIONAL RESEARCH

Finding information about research in medical education can be difficult. Educational research uses methods from the social sciences, including education, anthropology and social science. Educational research also uses many, varied statistical methods,[21] many of which are unfamiliar to healthcare professionals, who are more used to comparative statistics between two groups. Educational research uses methods that are rooted both in positivist (hypothesis testing) and in interpretivist (hypothesis generating) paradigms.
    Thus educational research uses a variety of methods. Choosing and using the best method for the particular research questions that are being asked depends on what you are trying to achieve.

Surveys: using questionnaires[22]

There are several advantages of using a questionnaire for educational research. It is feasible and economical in terms of time and effort to collect a range of views, from the whole population to be studied, rather than sampling just some parts of the population. The questionnaire data (especially for closed rating scale questions) may be analysed using statistical testing for significance and associations between different data, including data reduction techniques such as factor analysis.[21] Statistical testing to assess the reliability of the data uses techniques such as test–retest reliability using kappa, Wilcoxon signed-rank test and repeated-measures ANOVA, and internal consistency using Cronbach's alpha.
    The questionnaire may allow a search for new patterns by either of two methods:

1 open-ended questions, and free comments, analysed by qualitative methods – from which you may obtain the 'gem' of information that may be missed by closed questions[23]
2 principal-component factor analysis – a data reduction method that reduces the quantitative data from the Likert questions to a small number of factors with common characteristics.

The disadvantages of the questionnaire method include the common problem that pre-coded responses may not be sufficiently comprehensive to accommodate all answers, forcing the candidate to choose a view that does not accurately represent their own.[21] It is assumed that all respondents will understand the questions in the same way, and there is no way of clarifying the question. Non-response affects the quality of the data and thus the generalisability of the results, as responders may differ from non-responders.[24]

A questionnaire may thus be designed to include both open questions and space for free comments (to get at the gems), closed questions (yes/no questions, tick-box questions with specified categories), and scale items such as the Likert rating scale (points on a scale ranging from 'agree' to 'disagree').

Interviews

An interview has been defined as a 'two-person conversation initiated by the interviewer, for the purpose of gathering research-relevant information.'[22] It has several uses within educational research, as it can:
➤ gather information about the research questions
➤ develop ideas for new hypotheses
➤ be used in conjunction with other research methods
➤ validate, go deeper and explore new themes generated by other evaluation methods
➤ test hypotheses that have already been generated.

To ensure credibility and reliability, you should record, transcribe verbatim, and analyse interviews in detail.

Focus groups

The focus group is a form of group interview that utilises discussion and interaction between, ideally, four to eight group members.[25] The participants are encouraged to talk, exchange ideas, tell stories, comment on each others' ideas, and ask each other questions. This method is useful in evaluation to explore learners' knowledge and experiences, and to determine their views about the course. Focus groups should clarify ideas and views that might be less accessible in a one-to-one interview.

Kitzinger[25] gives advice on group composition, running the group, analysis and writing up focus-group-based research. It is essential that focus group activity is recorded and transcribed for detailed analysis. Digital recording using a boundary microphone (for 360-degree capture of what people say) will give a good sound quality and allows storage and electronic transfer of audio files to participants and colleagues for further comments.

Action research[22]

This is a technique that promotes change and improvement. It allows the researcher, as a participant in the project, to identify a problem, plan an intervention, put it into practice and study the outcome in depth as the project evolves. The researcher must study the subject that is being researched and reflect on the actions taken, and make detailed notes, recordings and critical analyses of meetings, interviews, focus groups and written materials. Action research involves cycles of strategic planning, action, observation and evaluation, and critical reflection on the results of the previous three steps. An example of this method in use was to design and run an improved induction to paediatrics for junior doctors.[26]

Controlled and comparative studies[22]

Many healthcare professionals will feel more familiar with controlled and comparative research designs. In experimental designs, a key feature is random allocation to groups (an experimental and a control group). In quasi-experimental designs, there is no random assignment, although there are two groups. For example, one group of students is taught in the 'normal' way and the other is taught by a new method, and the final assessment marks are compared.

Sometimes a natural experiment happens, and you may be fortunate enough to capture this. For example, when the quality of care points system was introduced into UK general practice, the performance of training practices versus non-training practices was investigated. Using practices matched for list size and deprivation scores, quality of care points were found to be significantly higher in training practices than in non-training practices.[27]

Other comparative studies include pre-test and post-test studies, and comparing cohorts over time.

Life history research

There has been a recent development of interest in educational research looking at narratives of teachers' lives, and life histories, and teachers' beliefs, in researching the teacher's viewpoints in a social and historical context.[28] It will include teachers' beliefs about their own identity. Identity is about how you see yourself, and also about how others see you. Your personal identity may not be the same as the one that others perceive you as having.

Life history research provides valuable insights into the way in which teachers comprehend their world and manage the constraints and conditions in which they work.[29] Teachers often import life history data into their accounts of classroom events. Life history research may be retrospective, where there is a reconstruction of past events from the present ideas and interpretations of the person concerned, or it may be contemporaneous, where the researcher endeavours to construct a description of an individual's life in progress at the present time. Often this research is undertaken using a series of in-depth interviews over time.

Mixed-methods studies

Combining various research methods within a study can be the best and most thorough way to examine your research question. For example, you may first conduct a series of interviews to obtain key concepts, and then use a questionnaire survey on a much larger group to test out these concepts.[30]

COMBINING TEACHING WITH RESEARCH

If you combine teaching with educational research, you can incorporate your research into your teaching. For example, research undertaken to establish what needs to be taught in a 'teaching the teachers' course (faculty development) supported choice of the content of the course.[30]

Research can help you to choose the most appropriate methods of evaluating your teaching (e.g. in the development of measurement tools to measure educational climate in the surgical operating room,[31] international validation of an educational climate tool[32] and demonstration of the effectiveness of teaching cross-cultural communication skills[33]).

Getting involved

How can you get involved with educational research? It may not be easy. It is important to undergo basic educational research methods training to prevent mistakes. Various textbooks address research methods in education – one highly regarded and comprehensive book is *Research Methods in Education*.[22]

Some university medical and dental education departments offer training courses, as does the Association for the Study of Medical Education (ASME). In some universities, the School of Education will run courses in educational research methods leading to a certificate or other award.

Find a senior mentor who is experienced in educational research, and who wishes to help you and pass on some of their expertise.

CONCLUSION

The implementation of best-evidence medical education is beset with difficulties. Educational interventions may be evaluated using the QUESTS dimensions:[8]

➤ the Quality of the research evidence (how reliable is it?)
➤ the Utility of the evidence (can the methods be adopted without modification?)
➤ the Extent of the evidence.
➤ the Strength of the evidence
➤ the Target or outcomes measured (how valid are they?)
➤ the Setting or context (how relevant is it?).

By evaluating innovations along these dimensions you may be able to improve your teaching, improve the learners' performance and have an impact on the better healthcare of your patients.

REFERENCES

1 Hart I. Best evidence medical education. *Med Teacher.* 1999; **21:** 453–4.
2 Edwards T. All the evidence shows . . . reasonable expectations of educational research. *Oxford Rev Educ.* 2000; **26:** 299–311.
3 Blunkett D. *Influence or Irrelevance: can social science improve government?* London: Department for Education and Employment. Reprinted in *Res Intelligence.* 2000; **March:** 12–21.
4 Pirrie A. Evidence-based practice in education: the best medicine. *Br J Educ Stud.* 2001; **49:** 124–36.

5 Hargreaves D. In defence of research for evidence-based teaching: a rejoinder to Martyn Hammersley. *Br Educ Res J.* 1997; **23**: 405–19.

6 Hammersley M. Educational research and a response to David Hargreaves. *Br Educ Res J.* 1997; **23**: 141–61.

7 Harden RM, Lilley PM. Best evidence medical education: the simple truth. *Med Teacher.* 2000; **22**: 117–19.

8 Harden RM, Grant J, Buckley G *et al.* BEME Guide No. 1. Best evidence medical education. *Med Teacher.* 1999; **21**: 553–62.

9 Harden RM, Lever R, Dunn WR *et al.* An experiment involving tape/slide programmes for lectures. *Lancet.* 1969; **1**: 933–5.

10 Gibbs G. Research into student learning. In: Smith B, Brown S, eds. *Research, Teaching and Learning in Higher Education.* London: Kogan Page; 1995.

11 Norman GR. Reflections on BEME. *Med Teacher.* 2000; **22**: 141–4.

12 Sackett DL, Wennberg JE. Choosing the best research design for each question. *BMJ.* 1997; **315**: 1636.

13 Chambers R, Boath E, Rogers D. *Clinical Effectiveness and Clinical Governance Made Easy.* 3rd edn. Oxford: Radcliffe Publishing; 2004.

14 Bligh J, Anderson MB. Medical teachers and evidence. *Med Educ.* 2000; **34**: 162–3.

15 Davies P. Approaches to evidence-based teaching. *Med Teacher.* 2000; **22**: 14–21.

16 Aspegren K. BEME Guide No. 2. Teaching and learning communication skills in medicine – a review with quality grading of articles. *Med Teacher.* 1999; **21**: 563–70.

17 Ebbert JO, Montori VM, Schultz J. The journal club in postgraduate medical education: a systematic review. *Med Teacher.* 2001; **23**: 455–61.

18 Hammick M. Interprofessional education: evidence from the past to guide the future. *Med Teacher.* 2000; **22**: 461–7.

19 Ten Cate O. What happens to the student? The neglected variable in educational outcome research. *Adv Health Sci Educ.* 2001; **6**: 81–8.

20 Belfield CR, Thomas HR, Bullock AD *et al.* Measuring effectiveness for best evidence medical education: a discussion. *Med Teacher.* 2001; **23**: 164–70.

21 Field A. *Discovering Statistics Using SPSS for Windows.* 2nd edn. London: Sage Publications; 2005.

22 Cohen L, Manion L, Morrison K. *Research Methods in Education.* 6th edn. London: Routledge; 2007.

23 Coffey A, Atkinson P. *Making Sense of Qualitative Data.* Thousand Oaks, CA: Sage Publications Inc.; 1996.

24 Bowling A. *Research Methods in Health.* Buckingham: Open University Press; 1997.

25 Kitzinger J. Introducing focus groups. In: Mays N, Pope C, eds. *Qualitative Research in Health Care.* London: BMJ Publishing Group; 1996.

26 Melville C, Wall DW, Samuels M. Resuscitating paediatric induction: an action research approach. *Med Educ.* 2001; **35**: 800–2.

27 Houghton G, Wall D, Norton B *et al.* Do GP training practices achieve higher QOF points? A study of the Quality and Outcomes Framework in Birmingham and the Black Country. *Educ Prim Care.* 2006; **17**: 557–71.

28 Syrjälä L, Estola E. *Telling and Re-Telling Stories as a Way to Construct Teachers' Identities and to Understand Teaching.* Paper presented at the European Conference on Educational Research, 22–25 September 1999, Lahti, Finland. www.leeds.ac.uk/educol/documents/00001311.htm

29 Goodson IF. Studying the teacher's life and work. *Teaching Teacher Educ.* 1994; **10**: 29–37.

30 Wall DW, McAleer S. Teaching the consultant teachers: setting the key content. *Med Educ.* 2000; **34**: 131–8.

31 Nagraj S, Wall D, Jones E. The development and validation of the mini-surgical theatre educational environment measure. *Med Teacher.* 2007; **29**: e192–7.

32 Wall D, Clapham M, Riquelme A *et al.* Is PHEEM a multi-dimensional instrument? An international perspective. *Med Teacher.* 2009; **31**: e521–7.

33 Chudley S, Skelton J, Wall D *et al.* Teaching cross-cultural communication skills: a course for UK and internationally trained general practice registrars. *Educ Prim Care.* 2007; **18**: 602–15.

FURTHER READING

- The 'best evidence in medical education' series in the *Medical Teacher* journal.
- Centre for Evidence Based Medicine: www.cebm.net
- BEME Collaboration: www.bemecollaboration.org
- Research Essential Skills in Medical Education (RESME) course: www.amee.org/index. asp?lm=96

Index